NPS STUDY GUIDE 2019-2020

NPS Exam Prep and Practice Test Questions for the
Neonatal and Pediatric Respiratory Care Exam

TABLE OF CONTENTS

ABOUT TRIVIUM TEST PREP

Trivium Test Prep uses industry professionals with decades worth of knowledge in the fields they have mastered, proven with degrees and honors in law, medicine, business, education, military, and more to produce high-quality test prep books such as this for students.

Our study guides are specifically designed to increase ANY student's score, regardless of his or her current scoring ability. At only 25% - 35% of the page count of most study guides, you will increase your score, while significantly decreasing your study time.

HOW TO USE THIS GUIDE

This guide is not meant to reteach you material you have already learned or waste your time on superfluous information. We hope you use this guide to focus on the key concepts you need to master for the test and develop critical test-taking skills. To support this effort, the guide provides:

- Practice questions with worked-through solutions
- Key test-taking tactics that reveal the tricks and secrets of the test
- Simulated one-on-one tutor experience
- Organized concepts with detailed explanations
- Tips, tricks, and test secrets revealed

Because we have eliminated "filler" or "fluff", you will be able to work through the guide at a significantly faster pace than other prep books. By allowing you to focus ONLY on those concepts that will increase your score, study time is more effective and you are less likely to lose focus or get mentally fatigued.

CRITICAL CARE

Respiratory therapists care for a large number of neonates and other children who are in need of critical care. This section includes the information you need to know in order to perform assessment, care planning, implementation, and evaluation of this critical care.

EVALUTING PERTINENT INFORMATION

THE HEALTH HISTORY

The purpose of the health history, within the context of pediatric data, is to elicit data and information relating to the mother's current and past states of health, illness, and wellness, because it can impact on the child's overall health and wellbeing. This maternal history is most significant immediately after birth and becomes progressively less significant as the child ages.

HEALTH HISTORY DATA

Data related to the patient, family members, and significant others is collected during the assessment phase. This data is also organized, validated with the patient and others, and documented.

Data can be primary or secondary. Primary data is provided by the patient themselves; secondary data is collected from other sources, such as previous medical records, laboratory test results, and radiographic studies.

Data can also be classified as subjective and objective. Subjective data is not measurable or observable, and it typically consists of the patient's own words. For example, a statement from the patient about their labor pain is subjective data. Objective data, on the other hand, is empirically measurable and observable. Vital signs, for example, are objective data.

Lastly, data can be quantitative or qualitative. Quantitative data consists of numbers; qualitative data consists of words. The amount of sodium or potassium in the patient's blood is quantitative; the patient's beliefs and perceptions are qualitative data.

During the interview process, the respiratory therapist must establish trust, inform the patient and their significant others about the purpose of the health history, ensure patient confidentiality, and maintain patient privacy and a comfortable environment.

Open-ended questions and closed-ended questions are used. Open-ended questions elicit full and meaningful answers from the patient that reflect the patient's own beliefs, knowledge, and feelings; closed-ended questions do not elicit the same richness of information. Closed-ended questions simply elicit a "no" or "yes" response and no other information. An example of an open-ended question is "Tell me about your child's shortness of breath." An example of a closed-ended question is "Has your child been exposed to the flu?"

PERFORMING THE HEALTH HISTORY

The health history consists of:

- *Demographic/biographical data*
- *Chief complaint*
- *Past medical history*
- *Current medical history and illness*
- *Family medical history*
- *Cultural history*
- *Spiritual history*
- *Lifestyle choices*
- *Social data*
- *Psychological status*
- *Patterns of health care*
- *Medication history*
- *Do not resuscitate status*
- *Previous patient education*

DEMOGRAPHIC AND BIOGRAPHICAL DATA

Biographical and demographic data is collected during the health history:

- *Name*
- *Address*
- *Telephone Number*
- *Emergency Contact Info*
- *Age*
- *Gender*
- *Marital status*

- *Occupation or Avocation (Hobby)*
- *Cultural Values and Beliefs*
- *Spiritual/Religious Preference(s)*
- *Health Insurance*
- *Patient's Access to Healthcare Services in the Community*

CHIEF COMPLAINT

This data is elicited from the patient by asking a question such as, "What brought you to the office today?" These types of questions should be open-ended. The responses to these questions will reflect the patient's perception of their current situation. Please note: The patient's response may or may not be accurate, but nonetheless, these perceptions are helpful.

PAST MEDICAL HISTORY

Past medical history includes:

- *Immunization status*

- *Childhood illnesses*

- *Chronic illnesses*

- *Genetic and congenital disorders*

- *Past injuries and accidents*

- *Possible exposures to environmental risk factors*

- *Dietary patterns*

- *Exercise patterns*

- *Current medications including over-the-counter medications, herbs, and supplements*

- *Substance use including illicit drugs and substances like caffeine and alcohol*

- *Prior surgical procedures*

- *Previous hospitalizations*

- *Allergies (medications, foods, environmental sources)*

- *Previous healthcare adverse events like medication toxicities and the adverse effects of anesthesia*

- *The number of live term births*

- *The number of preterm infants*

- *Number of pregnancies with abortion (therapeutic and spontaneous)*

- *Number of living children*

- *Prior pregnancy complications*

- *Prior deliveries in terms of neonatal weight, general level of development, and Apgar scores*

- *Psychosocial responses to previous pregnancies*

- *Psychosocial history related to depression, social support systems and any history of domestic violence*

FAMILY MEDICAL HISTORY

The family medical history includes data relating to:

- *Genetic and congenital disorders*

- *Diabetes*

- *Heart disease*

- *The presence of any chronic or acute psychosocial disorders*

- *The ages and the current state of health of grandparents, parents, siblings, and children*

- *The age and cause of death for grandparents, parents, siblings, and children*

CULTURAL HISTORY

Some of the cultural data collected during this phase of the health history include the person's ethnic and cultural customs, beliefs, practices and preferences.

SPIRITUAL HISTORY

Some of the data collected during this phase of the health history include the person's religious and spiritual customs, beliefs, practices, and preferences.

LIFESTYLE CHOICES

The respiratory therapist collects this data and information in order to identify possible risk factors and to provide a foundation for future teaching and health promotion activities:

- *Diet, including any dietary restrictions, the quality and quantity of food consumed, cultural preferences, and religious modifications*

- *Consumption patterns in relationship to illicit drugs, alcohol, and tobacco*

- *Sleep and rest patterns*

- *Exercise*

- *Occupational and avocational preferences*

- *Sociocultural Data*

Examples of sociocultural data are economic status, level of education, employment, family composition, support systems (such as family members, friends and community-based resources), income levels, home and neighborhood situations and conditions (including environmental and safety risks, social norms, and the accessibility of health care and public transportation.)

PSYCHOLOGICAL STATUS

Some of the psychological data collected during the health history include things like the patient's:

- *Attitude, mood, affect, thought processes, and coherence*

- *Coping skills and mechanisms and their successes or failures*

- *Stress and stressors*

- *Communication patterns*

- *Any history of a chronic or acute psychological disorder, such as depression, abuse, neglect, violence, apathy, suicidal thoughts, and panic disorders*

PATTERNS OF HEALTH CARE

The purpose of eliciting data and information about the patient's patterns of health care is to determine what type of healthcare resources they utilize. For example, does the patient use a primary care physician, a community clinic, specialists, etc.? Are these resources adequate for and accessible to the patient?

MEDICATION HISTORY

Medication reconciliation and the patient's medication history is one of the most important aspects of the admission process. Simply stated, medication reconciliation is a systematic and formal process for creating the most accurate list possible of a patient's current medications, and comparing this list to the medications ordered in the patient's medical record. For obvious reasons, all prescription medications, vitamins, over-the-counter medications, herbal remedies, nutritional and dietary supplements, vaccinations, blood derivatives, diagnostic and contrast agents, and radioactive medications are included in this list. The five steps of the formal medication reconciliation process are as follows:

1. *Generate and document a list of current medications*

2. *Generate a list of newly prescribed medications*

3. *Compare and contrast the two lists*

4. *Employ critical thinking and professional judgments during the comparison*

5. *Document the new list of medications and communicate with appropriate healthcare providers*

The Institute of Medicine's *Preventing Medication Errors* reports that greater than 40 percent of medication errors are the result of both the lack of medication reconciliation and the lack of communication and documentation when the patient is admitted, transferred, and discharged. Medication errors are a very commonly occurring medical error that can, and should be, prevented.

The primary purpose of medication reconciliation is to avoid a number of different errors including those related to omissions, faulty dosages, incorrect timing, duplications, drug-drug interactions, and adverse interactions between the current illness and a current medication.

Although medical doctors, the pharmacy, and the nursing department are often most typically and directly involved in this medication reconciliation process, respiratory therapists should review and verify this list, particularly in terms of respiratory care medications and medications that may adversely affect the patient's respiratory status.

DO NOT RESUSCITATE STATUS (DNR) AND OTHER END-OF-LIFE ISSUES

All patients should have end-of-life decisions, including whether they desire to be resuscitated, documented prior to the end of their life.

Advance care planning encompasses the DNR status, as well as a durable power of attorney for health care or health care surrogate, a living will, advance medical care directives, and a patient-completed values history. Most often, the advance medical care directive consists of both the living will and the durable power of attorney for health care. Ideally, all of these decisions and documents should be finished when the patient is competent and healthy. A durable power of attorney for health care, also referred to as a healthcare proxy or healthcare surrogate, is a legally appointed person who will make decisions relating to healthcare when the patient is not competent and able to give legal consent.

Advance medical care directives, also referred to as living wills and advance directives, contain the wishes of the patient in terms of treatments and interventions that they do and do not want carried out when they are no longer able to competently provide these consents and rejections of treatment.

The most commonly seen components of advance directives include choices relating to life support measures, mechanical ventilation, intravenous solution administration, and methods of artificial feeding, like tube feedings. Many patients at the end of life choose DNR and specifically state that they do not want mechanical ventilation, intravenous fluids and/or tube feedings.

These directives should be as specific and complete as possible. When an unanticipated event or treatment occurs that is not included in these advance directive, decisions are made by the durable power of attorney for healthcare in the best interests of the patient and their values.

Values histories further support the patient's beliefs and opinions in terms of healthcare decisions when decisions must be made and they have not already been anticipated and documented in the person's living will, and the durable power of attorney for healthcare needs guidance to make these unanticipated decisions. For example, has the patient expressed feelings about life without pain? Has the patient expressed beliefs about wanting to "die with dignity?" Although many patients do not have a values history, it is strongly recommended that healthcare professionals help the patient to complete one.

PREVIOUS PATIENT EDUCATION

Although data relating to previous patient education should be determined, previous patient education does not necessarily mean that patient and family members have achieved and maintained the knowledge, skills, and abilities that were addressed in the previous patient educational activity. For example, barriers to learning may have negatively impacted the success of this previous education, and the knowledge or skill that was addressed may have been forgotten. For these reasons, among others, all healthcare professionals must establish the patient and family members' baseline level of knowledge in order to plan future patient educational activities that meet these needs.

OTHER PERTINENT DATA

Other pertinent data include:

- *Admission notes*
- *Patient diagnosis*
- *Progress notes*
- *Respiratory care orders*

Admission Notes

All healthcare providers, including respiratory care professionals, must review the admission notes that are documented upon first contact or admission to a healthcare facility. These provide the patient's current state of illness, or disease, and a brief description of the progression of the illness that led to the current admission. Of particular importance are the medical notes, nursing notes and respiratory therapy notes. Pharmacy and dietary admission notes may also be reviewed, as indicated.

Progress Notes

Like admission notes, progress notes should also be reviewed on a regular basis. At times these notes should be reviewed on an hourly or more frequent basis when the patient's condition is unstable and frequently changing; if the patient's condition is relatively stable, these notes should be reviewed every shift.

Respiratory Care Orders

Respiratory therapists must be thoroughly aware of all current orders relating to respiratory care, not only upon initial patient contact but throughout the course of treatment and care. Like progress notes, there are occasions when these orders should be reviewed on an hourly or more frequent basis when the patient's condition is unstable and frequently changing.

Diagnoses

Diagnoses should be reviewed and integrated into the care of the patient throughout the course of treatment. Medical diagnoses reflect the specific diseases or illnesses that are currently causing the patient's signs and symptoms. Medical diagnoses can include both primary medical diagnoses and existing comorbidities. For example, patients may be admitted with the diagnosis of pulmonary embolism, but they may also be affected with heart disease or peripheral vascular disease. Comorbidities impact on the patient's current physical status, and they also alert healthcare professionals to potential complications and challenges in terms of treatment.

Medical diagnoses are based on the patient's medical history, the findings of a complete and thorough physical assessment and a number of different diagnostic tests. Medical diagnoses are not definitive when the signs are nonspecific to a disorder, or when symptoms are representative of a number of possible disorders that must be ruled out or eliminated.

Nursing diagnoses are different from medical diagnoses. The North American Nursing Diagnosis Association International (NANDA-I) is an association that develops and refines nursing diagnoses for the nursing profession. It provides a framework for standardized, consistent communication and nursing documentation. To read more about NANDA-I, visit the URL listed in the footnotes.

NEONATAL ASSESSMENT

The components of the neonate's physical status include:

- *The Apgar score*
- *Fetal lung development*
- *Fetal lung maturity*
- *Gestational age*
- *Neuromuscular maturity*
- *Physical maturity*
- *Head-to-toe physical assessment*

THE APGAR SCORE

Developed in the 1950s by Virginia Apgar, the Apgar score assesses a neonate's most basic physiological responses and adjustments to extrauterine life using five criteria. When this rapid assessment is done at one minute and, again, at five minutes after delivery, it makes rapid intervention and treatment possible when the neonate is not adequately adapting to extrauterine life.

The neonate's establishment of respiratory function after the cutting of the umbilical cord is the most critical adjustment. Ideally, air begins to inflate and adequately oxygenate the neonate with its first and subsequent respirations.

The neonate must also adequately adjust to circulatory changes immediately after the cutting of the umbilical cord and the expulsion of the placenta, which previously provided circulation to the neonate during intrauterine life. In response to extrautcrine life, for example, the neonate's ductus venosus, ductus arteriosus, and foramen ovale close.

The five criteria that the Apgar score uses to assess and measure neonate health can be easily remembered with the acronym APGAR, as follows:

A: *Appearance*

P: *Pulse*

G: *Grimace (Reflexes)*

A: *Appearance (Skin color)*

R: *Respirations*

Each of the criteria is scored as a 0, 1, or 2, then added up for an overall score between 0 and 10 (with 10 being the healthiest.)

1. *The Appearance or Skin Color:*

   0: The skin color is blue.

   1: The neonate's body is pink but the extremities are blue.

   2: The neonate's entire body is pink.

2. *The Heart Rate or Pulse (The pulse is assessed using a stethoscope):*

   0: The absence of a heartbeat.

   1: The pulse is less than 100 beats per minute (BPM.)

   2: The heart rate is more than 100 BPM.

3. *Grimace or Reflex Irritability in Response to a Mild Pinch Stimulus:*

0: No reaction whatsoever.

1: The neonate grimaces when it is stimulated.

2: Upon simulation, the neonate reacts, coughs, or cries.

4. *Muscle Tone or Activity:*

   0: The muscular tone is flaccid and floppy.

   1: The neonate has some, but fair, muscle tone.

   2: The neonate has active muscular activity and good tone.

5. *Respiratory Effort:*

   0: The absence of respiratory activity.

   1: The neonate has slow and irregular respiratory activity.

   2: The neonate has normal respiratory activity and it is able to cry well.

Although the Apgar scoring is done one minute after birth and then again in five minutes, it is done more often when the score remains abnormally low. An Apgar score of 7 or more is considered normal and it is indicative of good adaptation to extrauterine life; an Apgar score of 4 to 6 is considered low and indicative of moderate neonatal distress in response to extrauterine life; and an Apgar score of 3 or less is critically low and an indication of severe distress and poor neonatal status.

In most cases, a relatively low score immediately after delivery becomes near normal, or normal, five minutes after delivery. Apgar scoring is done and documented by nurses, doctors, and midwives.

A low score immediately after birth necessitates medical attention; however, it is not always an indication that serious long term problems are present in the newborn. On the other hand, there is a possibility that the neonate has serious neurological damage when the Apgar score remains less than 3 for more than 30 minutes after delivery. Scores less than 7 require immediate interventions and measures, such as physical stimulation to increase cardiac function, and oxygen supplementation, to facilitate the neonate's adjustment to extrauterine life. Some of the most commonly occurring causes of an Apgar score less than 7 are a difficult and prolonged labor and delivery process, a C section, and impaired respiratory functioning secondary to fluid in the airway.

A score of 10 is very rare because a majority of neonates lose 1 point for transient and temporary cyanotic extremities immediately after delivery. In fact, a score of 7 to 9 is indicative of good health for the neonate. When cyanosis does not resolve, however, a congenital cardiopulmonary anomaly or central nervous system (CNS) depression may be present.

FETAL LUNG DEVELOPMENT

Intrauterine lung development consists of the five stages, as below:

1. *Embryonic:* Major bronchi, diaphragm and trachea develop

2. *Pseudoglandular:* More airways develop; goblet cells appear

3. *Canalicular:* Respiratory acini and vascular bed develop

4. *Saccular:* Saccules become more complex and gas exchanging surface area increases

5. *Alveolar:* Alveoli develop

Lung development continues after birth and through childhood. For example, the number of alveoli, gas exchanging surface area and lung volume all increase. Some factors that impact pre/postnatal lung development are:

- *Altered metabolic states,* such as that which occurs with starvation, hypoxia and hyperoxia

- *Nutritional deprivation,* which can adversely affect lung structure, growth and functioning

- *The postnatal delivery of high oxygen concentrations,* which are toxic to developing pulmonary tissue

- *Oligohydramnios,* a low amount of amniotic fluid, that can lead to lung hypoplasia

- *A low respiratory rate,* which can lead to the lack of lung elasticity in the lung parenchyma

- *Hormonal and metabolic alterations,* which can lead to dysmorphic lungs, enlarged air spaces, and dilated alveolar ducts and saccules

- *Down's syndrome,* which leads to larger and fewer than normal postnatal alveoli

Commonly occurring abnormalities of the lung include pulmonary hypoplasia, malformed alveolar cell development, impaired surfactant production, and fetal lung liquid. Pulmonary hypoplasia is the failure of the fetal lung to develop in terms of sufficient cells, sufficient alveoli and sufficient airways. Lung compression prior to the 16th week of gestation is associated with pulmonary hypoplasia. Malformed alveolar cell development can affect the development of Type I and Type II pneumocytes, which create the permeable membrane for gas diffusion and the production of surfactant, respectively.

Surfactant decreases the surface tension in the alveoli, allowing the lung to perform without collapse. The components of surfactant are neutral lipids, phospholipids, and proteins. Fetal lungs produce about 300 mL of liquid per day to fill the airways. The balance between production and excretion into the amniotic sac or ingestion is essential to lung development. This fluid production comes from the fetal pulmonary, rather than the bronchial, circulation.

LUNG MATURITY

Lung maturation studies include measuring:

- *Lecithin/Sphingomyelin (L/S Ratio)*

- *Phosphatidylglycerol (PG)*
- *Lung profile*

The L/S Ratio

The L/S ratio, a measure of fetal lung maturity, is the amount of lecithin in comparison to the amount of sphingomyelin in the amniotic fluid. Fetal lungs need surfactant in order to properly function. Surfactant, which is composed of lecithin and sphingomyelin, lowers the alveolar surface tension so the alveoli are stabilized and a certain amount of air remains in the alveoli after expiration during extrauterine life.

The L/S ratio changes throughout the course of the pregnancy. Early in the pregnancy, the amount of lecithin in the amniotic fluid is less than the amount of sphingomyelin. At approximately the 20th week of gestation, the L/S ratio is about 0.5:1. Later, between 30th and 32nd weeks of gestation, the amounts are about the same, therefore, the L/S ratio is 1:1; similarly, by the 35th week of gestation, the amount of lecithin exceeds the amount of sphingomyelin. At this point, the L/S ratio is 2:1. A ratio of less than 2:1 is not normal and is an indicator that the neonate, when born, may be affected with Infant Respiratory Distress Syndrome (IRDS.) A ratio of less than 1.5 indicates that the patient is a high risk for IRDS, which is common in preterm neonates.

PG

PG is also found in surfactant. Normally, this phospholipid begins to appear at the 36th week of gestation and its level continues to rise during the duration of the pregnancy; however, when the mother is affected with conditions such as eclampsia, severe preeclampsia, premature rupture of the membranes, and diabetes, PG can be present before the 36th week of gestation, which signals the risk of IRDS. The complete absence of PG signals a high risk of IRDS.

Lung Profile

A lung profile consists of the combination of the L/S ratio and PG. Lung maturity is assessed and confirmed when the L/S ratio is 2:1 and PG is present.

GESTATIONAL AGE

The assessment of the neonate, in respect to gestational age, is done within two to twelve hours after the delivery of the neonate because gestational age and neonate weight are two major indicators of neonatal mortality and morbidity.

The New Ballard Scale is used for this gestational age assessment as the baseline against which the neonate's growth and development can be compared and monitored. The normal and expected parameters for the neonate in terms of physical measurements are as follows:

- *Length: 18-22" (45-55 cm)*

- *Weight: 2,500-4,000 g*

- *Chest Circumference: 12-13" (30-33 cm)*

- *Head Circumference: 12.6-14.5" (32 to 36.8 cm)*

The New Ballard Scale measures neuromuscular maturity and physical maturity. Ranges of development, depending on the specific assessment, can range from -1 to 5. The total score indicates the maturity rating in terms of the number of weeks of gestation. For example, a total score of 35 indicates that the neonate is at 38 weeks of gestation.

MEASURING NEONATAL NEUROMUSCULAR MATURITY

Assessment	Description	Range
Posture	Posture from fully extended to fully flexed	0 to 4
Arm Recoil	A spontaneous return to flexion when the arm is passively extended by the assessor	0 to 4

Scarf Sign	The crossing of the arms over the chest	-1 to 4
Square Window Formation	The movement of the neonate's wrist	-1 to 4
Heel to Ear Movement	The extent to which the neonate's heel can reach the ears	-1 to 4
Popliteal Angle	The extent, or angle, to which the neonate's knees can extend	-1 to 5

MEASURING NEONATAL PHYSICAL MATURITY

Assessment	Description	Range
Lanugo	The presence and amount of lanugo	-1 to 4
Plantar Surface Creases	The amount of creases on the neonate's sole from less than 40 mm to 50 mm	-1 to 4
Skin Texture	The texture of the neonate's skin ranging from sticky and transparent to wrinkled and cracked	-1 to 5
Development of the Genitalia	In males, the development of the scrotum and testes from smooth and flat to those that have deep rugae. In females, the development of the clitoris and labia from flat labia and a prominent clitoris, to the development of the labia majora, covering the labia minora and the clitoris	-1 to 4
Ear and Eyes	The extent to which the neonate's eyes	-1 to 4

	open and the ear cartilage is developed	
Amount of Breast Tissue	The extent to which the neonate's breasts are developed from flat to a 5 to 10 mm bud and a full areola	-1 to 4

After these assessments, the gestational age of the infant is determined and classified according to the neonate's weight, as follows:

- *Low birth weight:* Neonatal weight is less than 2,500g at time of delivery.

- *Appropriate for gestational age:* Neonatal weight ranges from 10th to 90th percentile.

- *Large for gestational age:* Neonatal weight is above the 90th percentile.

- *Small for gestational age:* Neonatal weight is below the 10th percentile.

- *Intrauterine growth restriction:* Growth not meeting expected norms.

Other classifications that are important in terms of gestational age include:

- *Term:* The neonate is born between the beginning of the 38th week of gestation and the end of the 42nd week of gestation.

- *Preterm:* The neonate is born before the end of the 37th week of gestation.

- *Post-term:* The neonate is born after the end of the 42nd week of gestation.

- *Post-mature:* The neonate is born after the end of the 42nd week of gestation and there is some evidence and signs of placental insufficiency.

To place gestational age into context, the estimated date of birth, or delivery, under normal circumstances is calculated using Nagle's rule. See an example below.

- *The First Day of the Last Menstrual Period: September 20th*

- *Subtract 3 Months: June 20th*

- *Add 7 Days: June 20th plus 7 days = June 27th*

- *Estimated Date of Delivery: June 27th of the following year*

THE HEAD-TO-TOE PHYSICAL ASSESSMENT

A thorough physical assessment can be done with the following components:

- *General survey*

- *Vital signs*

- *Oxygen saturation*

- *The integumentary system assessment*

- *The assessment of the head*

- *The assessment of the neck*

- *The assessment of the thorax and lungs*

- *Lung sounds*

- *The assessment of the cardiovascular system*

- *The assessment of the peripheral vascular system*

- *The assessment of the breast and axillae*

- *The assessment of the abdomen*

- *The assessment of the musculoskeletal system*

- *The assessment of the neurological system*

- *The assessment of the male and female genitalia and inguinal lymph nodes*

- *The assessment of the rectum and anus*

Four Basic Methods of Physical Assessment

The four basic methods or techniques that are used for physical assessment are:

1. *Inspection*   3. *Percussion*

2. *Palpation*   4. *Auscultation*

Inspection

Inspection is purposeful and systematic visual inspection and examination of the patient. It is typically the first aspect a head-to-toe assessment.

Palpation

The palpation technique employs the sense of touch. Palpation can be categorized, or classified, as light and deep. Light palpation is used more often because deep palpation must be used with caution. To palpate, the RT applies their fingertips to the patient's body to assess temperature, mobility, degree of distention, pain points, texture, position, size, symmetry, tenderness, any vibrations, pulses, and the presence of abnormalities like masses or asymmetry.

Percussion

Percussion is used to assess the size and shape of internal organs and tissue, as well as assess underlying structures in terms of solidity, regularity/irregularity, and the presence or absence of fluid and air, for example.

Percussion is performed by striking the patient's body and assessing the sounds and vibrations produced. The two types of percussion are indirect and direct. The five types of sounds elicited during percussion are flatness, resonance, hyper-resonance, tympany, and dullness.

Flatness is normally assessed over muscles and bones; resonance is a hollow sound that is heard, for example, over the air-filled lungs; hyper-resonance is a booming sound that is heard over abnormal lung tissue, as occurs among patients with chronic obstructive pulmonary disease (COPD); tympany is heard over the stomach as a drum-like sound; and dullness is normally heard over solid organs, such as the spleen, heart, and liver. It is a thud-like sound.

Auscultation

Using a stethoscope, the assessor listens to sounds produced in the body. The four types of auscultated sound are pitch, duration, intensity, and quality.

Pitch is the frequency of vibrations, and can be high or low; duration is the length of time from the beginning to the end of the sound; intensity is characterized along a continuum from softness to loudness; quality includes subjective sound characteristics such as irregularity, regularity, grating, booming, and others.

The General Survey

The general survey is an overall look at the patient, their appearance and general state of health. Some of the components of this general survey are not performed on a neonate or infant. For example, gait and balance are assessed only on patients that can walk. Some things that the RT will assess as part of the general survey include:

- *Weight, height, and body build*

- *Posture, gait, and balance*

- *Hygiene and grooming*

- *The person's actual age as compared to how old they appear*

- *Oral and bodily odors*

- *Signs of distress and/or obvious signs of illness or deformity, such as dyspnea, swelling, and reddened skin*

Vital Signs

The vital signs include pulse, body temperature, respirations, blood pressure, and oxygen saturation, which is the newest of all the vital signs.

Pulse

Pulse can be assessed at a number of sites, including the apical area (using a stethoscope.) It can be assessed with the index and middle fingers near the radius, the temporal area of the head, the carotid area of the neck, in the femoral area of the groin, the lower legs behind the knee (popliteal), the inner aspect of the arm in the brachial area, the front of the foot (dorsalis pedis) and near the ankle (posterior tibial.) Pulses are assessed for rate, volume, intensity, rhythm, and bilateral equality. The parameters of a normal adult pulse are 80-100 BPM.

Neonates have different parameters dependent on their weight: For a small neonate (4.5-7 pounds) a normal resting heart rate is 120-160 BPM, and for larger neonates and infants, a normal resting pulse is 80-140. Like all children, neonates will experience a substantial increase in their heart rate when they are under significant stress, or if they have a fever.

Temperature

Body temperature results from the differences between heat production and heat losses. The normal oral bodily temperature is 98.6 degrees F, or 36.7 to 37 degrees centigrade. Temperature can be taken at a number of sites including the mouth, rectum, ear, and axillae.

The oral route is contraindicated among unconscious and uncooperative patients, infants, and small children. The ear is the preferred site for infants and young children. The rectal route is contraindicated when a patient is affected with a seizure disorder, heart disease, or any kind of rectal disorder.

Respirations

Respiratory rate is the only vital sign that humans have some conscious control over, at least until the point when carbon dioxide builds up in the body and one is forced to breathe. Respirations are assessed, and documented, in terms of rate, regularity, depth and quality, which can include some assessment findings like stridor, dyspnea, and shortness of breath. An increased respiratory rate can occur as the result of fear, anxiety, pain, acidosis, and a fever; a decreased respiratory rate can result from alkalosis, sedation, CNS depression, and a coma.

Blood Pressure

Blood pressure results from the pressure of blood flow as it moves through the arteries. The systolic blood pressure indicates the amount of pressure exerted on the arteries during the heart's contractions; the diastolic blood pressure indicates the pressure exerted on the arteries when the heart is at rest. Blood pressure is most often measured over the upper arm just above the antecubital space, although it can also be measured on other sites such as the legs.

Pulse pressure is defined as the mathematical difference between systolic and diastolic blood pressures. For example, a patient with a systolic blood pressure of 197 and a diastolic of 110 has a pulse pressure of 87.

Oxygen Saturation

Oxygen saturation reflects the amount of oxygen saturation in arterial blood. It is measured by placing a sensor on the person's finger. At times, the forehead, nose, or ear can be used for these measurements.

The Assessment of the Integumentary System

The integumentary consists of the hair, skin, fingernails and toenails. The hair is inspected and thoroughly assessed in terms of distribution, amount, the presence of any alopecia or baldness, hair thickness, and the presence of any abnormalities like an infestation or infection. Nails are assessed in terms of texture, blanching, and shape (curvature and angle.) The skin around the nails is also observed, as well as the color of the nail beds. The skin is assessed with inspection and palpation and the components of this assessment include the skin's color, moisture, turgor, temperature, and the presence of any edema and/or skin lesions.

The Assessment of the Head

The assessment of the head consists of these areas:

Face and Skull

The face and facial expressions are inspected for abnormities and a lack of symmetry, both which may indicate neurological damage such as that which occurs with a cerebrovascular accident. The skull is assessed for shape, size, and symmetry, and the presence or absence of any tenderness, nodules, or depressions are also noted.

Nose and Sinuses

The external nose is assessed for its size, shape, color, symmetry, and the presence of any nasal flaring and/or discharge. The interior nasal passages are assessed for intactness and patency, the presence of any masses, and any abnormalities of the cartilaginous and/or bone tissue. The frontal and maxillary sinuses are assessed for any tenderness.

Eyes and Vision

The assessor examines the conjunctiva, the lacrimal glands and ducts, the clarity of the corneas, the eyelashes, eyebrows, eyebrow movement, eye movement, blinking, and the pupils for color, shape, size, symmetry of size, accommodation and reactions to light. Visual acuity is assessed using the Snellen chart.

The eyes are also inspected for signs of infection and irritation such as discharge, redness or hollowness. They are also assessed for abnormalities such as a sunken or protruding appearance.

The Ears and Hearing

The ear structures and the sense of hearing are assessed with this portion of the physical assessment. The earlobes, or auricles, are assessed in terms of symmetry, texture, position, color, elasticity, and any areas of tenderness. The tympanic membrane is examined for intactness and color. The external ear canal is assessed in terms of the amount of cerumen, and the presence of any blood, pus, abnormal structures, and/or lesions.

In order to test for gross hearing, the patient is asked to listen and respond by telling if they hear both whispered and normal words. Bone conduction is assessed using Weber's test. The Rinne test compares air conduction to the bone conduction. A tuning fork is needed to perform these two tests.

Mouth and Throat

The lips are assessed for color, texture, and symmetry; missing, loose and damaged teeth are noted (this is not applicable to neonates for obvious reasons); the gums are assessed for color and the presence of any sores or other lesions; the cheeks, or buccal membranes, and the inner lips are assessed for moisture, and the presence of any lesions.

The color, movement, and presence of any lesions are assessed on the tongue and all of its surfaces. In order to perform this assessment, the patient sticks their tongue out while the assessor pulls it forward using a dry gauze pad.

The soft and hard palates are assessed for color, texture and the presence of any lesions; the salivary glands are examined for swelling or redness; the uvula is assessed for position, movement and color. Lastly, the gag reflex is checked and the tonsils and oropharynx are assessed for size, color, and the presence of any lesions or swelling while using a penlight and tongue blade.

The Assessment of the Neck

The assessment of the neck consists of these areas:

The Thyroid Gland

This butterfly-shaped gland is inspected for symmetry, movement during swallowing, and the presence of any lesions or masses. The thyroid gland is auscultated for bruits and is additionally palpated in order to determine its size and smoothness.

Neck Muscles

The neck muscles are assessed by observing head movements, muscular strength, and observing for the presence of any swelling or masses.

Lymph Nodes and Trachea Deviation

The entire neck area is palpated for any lymph node swelling. Additionally, any deviation of the trachea from normal centrality of position is noted.

The Assessment of the Thorax and Lungs

The assessor examines the lateral, posterior, and anterior thorax, for size, shape, symmetry, and any signs of spinal misalignment and abnormality. The posterior chest is palpated for fremitus and respiratory excursion; the thorax is percussed, using a zigzag pattern. To assess the lungs, diaphragmatic movement is visually assessed and the chest is auscultated for breath sounds.

Lung and Breath Sounds

The normal breath sounds are:

1. *Bronchovesicular*

   These are heard during both inspiration and expiration between the scapulae and between the 1st and 2nd intercostal spaces.

2. *Vesicular*

   These are best heard during inspiration over the base of the lungs or over the peripheral lung area.

The abnormal, or adventitious, breath sounds are:

3. *Tubular or Bronchial*

   Tubular, or bronchial, breath sounds have a shorter inspiratory phase than expiratory phase. They are louder than vesicular sounds and it is NOT normal to hear these sounds over normal lung tissue.

4. *Wheezing*

   Wheezes are squeaky, high-pitched breath sounds that are most typically heard during expiration. They can be heard over all lung fields. Coughing does not diminish or decrease wheezing like it does with rhonchi. Tumors and other forms of enlargement, such as occurs with swelling, create secretions that can lead to adventitious breath sounds.

5. *Gurgles or Rhonchi*

These sounds are harsh, low pitched, and gurgling in nature. They are produced when airways are narrowed by such abnormalities as tumors, swelling, or secretions. They are heard most often over the trachea and the bronchi. Gurgles can be diminished when the patient coughs.

6. *Rales (Crackles)*

Rales, or crackles, are most often heard over the bases of the lungs. This is similar to the sound that can be created by rolling a small amount of hair next to your ear. They are fine, short, crackling sounds produced when fluid or mucus is present in a lung passage.

7. *Friction Rub*

Friction rub sounds are grating. They occur when the pleural surfaces are inflamed and rubbing together. These can be heard during both the inspiratory and expiratory phases of respiration and are most often over the lateral or lower anterior chest. These sounds can indicate an infection affecting the heart.

8. *Stridor*

Stridor is a squeaking, high pitched sound upon inspiration resulting from a large upper respiratory airway obstruction. It closely mimics the sound of wheezing, so the assessor should use a stethoscope over the neck – if the sound is louder in this area, it is more likely stridor than wheezing.

The Assessment of the Cardiovascular System

Cardiovascular assessment, in addition to vital signs, includes:

- *Inspection*
- *Palpation*
- *Auscultation*

<u>Heart Sounds</u>

Heart sounds occur as the result of the heart valves opening and closing. Heart sounds are classified and characterized as systolic and diastolic.

The systolic heart sounds are:

- *S_1 or the first heart sound*
- *Clicks*

S_1 in combination with S_2, which is a diastolic heart sound, are the normal heart sounds that we hear as "lub-dub." S_1 begins when systole begins and results from primarily mitral valve closure, but it can occur to a lesser extent by tricuspid valve closure. This heart sound may be high pitched and split; however, when it is loud, it can indicate mitral stenosis; with mitral regurgitation, it can be absent or soft sounding. It is normally asynchronous because left ventricular systole occurs slightly before right ventricular systole.

Clicks are only heard at different phases of systole. They can be singular or multiple and are differentiated from S_1 and S_2 heart sounds with their briefer duration and higher pitch. Congenital pulmonic stenosis, aortic stenosis and severe pulmonary hypertension are marked with clicks at the very beginning of S_1. It is believed that these clicks occur as the result of abnormal ventricular wall tension. Clicks that occur during the middle or later phases of systole are heard among patients affected with tricuspid or mitral valve prolapse, and it is believed that these clicks occur as the result of abnormally high tension against valve leaflets, or an elongated chordae tendonae.

The diastolic heart sounds are:

1. *S_2*
2. *S_3*
3. *S_4*
4. *Diastolic knocks*
5. *Mitral valve sounds*

Diastolic heart sounds are of lower pitch, softer, and longer in duration than the systolic heart sounds. S_2 is the only normal diastolic sound, except in rare cases. S_2, which begins at the beginning of diastole, is heard when the pulmonic and aortic valves close; the aortic valve typically closes prior to the closure of the pulmonic valve closure with the exception of occasions where the aortic valve closes late or the pulmonic valve closes early. The former often occurs with the presence of aortic stenosis or left bundle branch block cardiac arrhythmia; the latter often occurs when the patient is affected with a pre-excitation disorder. Additionally, a late pulmonic valve closure can occur as the result of an increase of blood flow through the right ventricle, as occurs with an atrial septal defect, or complete right bundle branch block.

S_3, when it occurs, is heard early during diastole at the time when the heart's ventricle is dilated and not compliant. It can indicate serious abnormal ventricular functioning among adult patients, though in rare cases, it is normal among pregnant women, some children, and adults up to about 40 years of age.

Right ventricular problems are signaled when the S_3 heart sound is heard best, and only during inspiration when the patient is in the supine position; left ventricular S_3 is best heard during expiration and when the patient is in the left lateral decubitus position.

The S_4 heart sound is heard best using the bell of the stethoscope; it typically indicates less ventricular dysfunction than an S_3 heart sound. During inspiration, the right ventricle S_4 heart sound increases and the left ventricle S_4 heart sound decreases. S_4 heart sounds are most typically found after a myocardial infarction and with myocardial ischemia. S_4 heart sounds without any S_3 heart sounds occur most often in diastolic left ventricular dysfunction; S_3 heart sounds accompanied with S_4 heart sounds are typically found among patients affected with systolic left ventricular dysfunction.

A diastolic knock, when present, occurs during the early diastolic phase. It is characterized as a thudding loud sound that results from an abrupt cessation of ventricular filling as the result of a constricting and noncompliant pericardium.

Mitral valve opening snaps, often heard during early diastole when the patient is affected with mitral and/or tricuspid stenosis, are short, high-pitched sounds best auscultated with the stethoscope's diaphragm, although, at times, they can be heard at the heart's apex. The greater and more severe the mitral stenosis, the closer any opening snap will be to the pulmonic aspect of S_2. Snap sounds are loudest when valve leaflets remain somewhat elastic but they progress to soft sounds and then to their disappearance when fibrosis, calcification, and/or sclerosis of the valve occurs.

Murmurs

Murmurs are of longer duration than heart sounds, and can be characterized as systolic, diastolic, or continuous. They are also characterized by their location and are graded according to their intensity as below.

1. *Barely audible*

2. *Soft but easily audible*

3. *Loud but without a thrill*

4. *Loud and with a thrill*

5. *Loud and audible with minimal stethoscope chest contact*

6. *Loud and audible without stethoscope chest contact*

Murmur timing provides information about its cause and etiology:

Timing of the Murmur	Cause of the Murmur
A mid systolic ejection murmur	• Obstruction of the aorta • Pulmonic obstruction • Dilation of the ascending aorta or the pulmonary artery • Increased flow across the aortic or pulmonic valve
A mid to late systolic murmur	• Papillary muscle impairment • Mitral valve prolapse
A holosystolic murmur	• A ventral septal defect

	• Regurgitation of the tricuspid or mitral valve
An early diastolic regurgitant murmur	• Regurgitation of the aortic valve or the mitral valve • A congenital abnormality of the bicuspid valve with or without the presence of a ventricular septal defect • The Tetralogy of Fallot • A dilation of the valve ring as that which occurs with Marfan syndrome and pulmonary hypertension
A mid diastolic murmur	• Mitral stenosis and/or regurgitation • Patent ductus arteriosus • Complete heart block • A ventricular or atrial septal defect • Tricuspid stenosis or regurgitation • Atrial tumors or thrombi
A continuous heart murmur	• An aortic septal defect • Patent ductus arteriosus • Pulmonary artery coarctation • Multiple other causes

Pericardial friction rubs are high-pitched, scratchy sounds occurring when the pericardial sac rubs during contractions. It is heard best with the stethoscope's diaphragm when the patient is in an upright position and leaning forward. This sound is associated with infiltrations, infections and inflammations such as pericarditis.

Sinus Bradycardia

Sinus bradycardia occurs when the SA node takes longer than normal to depolarize as the result of some parasympathetic stimulation. The duration of diastole increases while the cardiac output decreases. This arrhythmia is often found among patients affected with coronary artery disease, during a myocardial infarction, secondary to increased intracranial pressure, and the result of some medications, such as digitalis and beta-blockers. Some of the general signs and symptoms of bradycardia are:

- *Fainting*
- *Weakness*
- *Dizziness*
- *Fatigue*

- *Shortness of breath*
- *Chest pain*
- *Confusion*

The treatment depends on the type of electrical conduction problem, the severity of symptoms, and the cause.

Sinus Tachycardia

Sinus tachycardia is associated with sympathetic nervous system stimulation, such as occurs with strenuous exercise, stress, pain, hyperthyroidism, caffeine use, and a cardiovascular response to hypovolemia and hypotension. Some of the general signs and symptoms of tachycardia are:

- *Palpitations*
- *Chest pressure or tightness*

- *Dizziness*
- *Lightheadedness*

Like sinus bradycardia, the treatment of sinus tachycardia depends on the type of electrical conduction problem, the severity of symptoms, and the cause. Sinus bradycardia and sinus tachycardia both have all the features of a normal sinus rhythm, other than a normal rate of from 60 to 100 BPM.

Atrial Flutter

Atrial flutter occurs during rapid atrial depolarization. The cardiac rate may bc irregular, and the danger of thrombosis is present but not to the extent as with atrial fibrillation. Some causes of atrial flutter are heart failure, chronic pulmonary disease, and right-sided heart enlargement. It is treated with digitalis, beta-blockers, calcium channel blockers, amiodarone, and cardioversion.

Atrial Fibrillation

Atrial fibrillation is a relatively common arrhythmia among those affected with pulmonary embolus, hypoxia, mitral valve disorder, congestive heart disease, and among the elderly. Cardiac output is decreased with this dysrhythmia. Emergency cardioversion may be indicated immediately after the administration of heparin or low molecular weight heparin to prevent thromboembolism.

Premature Atrial Contractions

Premature atrial contractions occur as the result of atrial cells taking over the role of the SA node. Normal QRS complexes occur but are preceded by a premature P wave. This arrhythmia can result from nicotine use, fatigue, alcohol, digitalis, electrolyte imbalances, ischemia, and hypoxia.

Paroxysmal Supraventricular Tachycardia

With this arrhythmia, the atria or the AV junction takes over the pacemaker role from the body's natural pacemaker, which is the SA node. It usually appears and disappears in a rather rapid manner. Some of the causes of paroxysmal supraventricular tachycardia are nicotine, caffeine, alcohol, stress, electrolyte imbalances, hypoxic episodes, and ischemia.

This cardiac arrhythmia is sometimes short lived and self-limiting. Simple coughing or carotid massage may readily resolve it. Other treatment interventions include adenosine intravenously and cardioversion when the patient is unstable as a result of this dysrhythmia.

First-Degree Atrioventricular Block

First-degree atrioventricular block occurs when the AV node impulse is delayed, thus leading to a prolonged PR interval. The P wave is present before each QRS complex. It is very often asymptomatic, and treatment is typically not indicated unless the patient is symptomatic. However, it should be noted that first-degree atrioventricular blocks can lead to more severe types of heart block.

Second-Degree Atrioventricular Block, Type I

Second-degree atrioventricular (AV) block Type I is also referred to as Wenckebach and Mobitz Type I arrhythmias. This dysrhythmia is characterized by progressive delays of conduction through the AV node, which progressively lengthens the PR interval until it results in a missing QRS interval and a non-conducted P wave. Treatment may not be necessary unless the patient is symptomatic. Some cases may be caused by digoxin toxicity.

Second-Degree Atrioventricular Block, Type II

Second-degree AV block Type II, also referred to as Mobitz Type II, occurs when the AV node impulses are intermittently blocked and do not reach the heart's ventricles. Second-degree AV block Type II can lead to complete heart block. Treatment includes supplemental oxygen, intravenous atropine, and a temporary pacemaker.

Complete Heart Block (Third-Degree Heart Block)

Third-degree heart block, or complete AV disassociation, occurs when no atrial impulses reach the ventricle, so a ventricular or junctional pacemaker takes over. This causes a lack of coordination between the ventricles and the atria; the ventricular and atrial rates are different, and the QRS complex is wide.

Some of the risk factors associated with complete heart block are medications like beta-blockers and digoxin, a myocardial infarction, coronary heart disease, an atrial septal defect, and acute rheumatic fever. The signs and symptoms include an altered level of consciousness, syncope, and chest pain.

Emergency treatment is necessary. Cardiac failure and cardiac arrest can occur, so cardiac pacing should be immediately started, alongside preparation for life support.

Premature Ventricular Contractions

Premature ventricular contractions are also referred to as extra-systole, premature ventricular complexes, and premature ventricular ectopic beats. It is a life-threatening emergency. With this irregularity, ventricular irritability causes abnormal impulses from an ectopic area in the ventricle. This can be caused by electrolyte imbalances, acidosis, hypoxia, ischemia, and digitalis toxicity.

Premature ventricular contractions can occur in isolation (single focus) or in clusters (multifocal.) Multifocal patterns are called bigeminy and trigeminy, respectively, and couplets and triplets are two and three PVCs in succession, respectively.

Ventricular Tachycardia

No cardiac impulses come from the atrium with life threatening ventricular tachycardia. This arrhythmia often leads to ventricular fibrillation and asystole unless it is immediately treated. The QRS complex is broadened and the rate is dangerously fast and inefficient. Significant hemodynamic compromise occurs rapidly. Emergency interventions include cardioversion, intravenous lidocaine and magnesium sulfate, and antiarrhythmic medications, such as amiodarone.

Ventricular Fibrillation

Ventricular fibrillation occurs when there are chaotic and rapid signals from ectopic ventricular sites. All of the ventricular contractions are ineffective; therefore, no cardiac output occurs. Death is very likely when this arrhythmia persists for more than six minutes. The treatment involves immediate advanced life support, including defibrillation, intravenous adrenaline, and 100% supplemental oxygen. A lack of treatment leads to asystole.

Asystole

Asystole, or a flat line, is the total and complete absence of any ventricular activity, despite the fact that atrial impulses and P waves may be present. Immediate advanced life support is necessary. Intravenous adrenaline, sodium bicarbonate, atropine and 100% oxygen may help save the patient's life.

The Assessment of the Peripheral Vascular System

The peripheral vascular system is assessed by palpating the bilateral pulses to determine volume, equality, and other characteristics such as regularity. The carotid pulse is auscultated for bruits. The jugular veins are inspected for any signs of distention or abnormal pulsation while the patient is in the semi-Fowler's position.

The peripheral veins in the legs and arms are inspected for their general condition and for any signs of tenderness, swelling, phlebitis, particularly in the lower extremities. Perfusion is assessed by inspecting the color and temperature of the skin, which assesses the adequacy of blood flow.

The Assessment of the Breast and Axillae

During this phase of the physical assessment, the RT uses the surfaces of all fingertips and palpates the lymph nodes and the breasts for any tenderness or masses.

The breast and the axillae are assessed using both palpation and inspection, among both males and females. The breasts and the areola are assessed for shape, size, contour, color, and the presence or absence of any lumps, lesions, dimpling, retraction, swelling, edema, and/or hyperpigmentation. The nipples are examined for any discharge, which is an abnormal finding unless the female is lactating.

The Assessment of the Abdomen

The abdomen is inspected for size, movement, contour, size, movement, and skin integrity. Any fluid buildup, or ascites, and any aortic pulsations are abnormal. The abdomen is auscultated for the presence of bowel sounds in all four of the quadrants: upper right, upper left, lower right, and lower left. All four quadrants are also palpated, lightly at first, for any tenderness, guarding, or masses. Later, deep palpation determines the presence of the findings from light palpation. The bladder is also palpated to assess for urinary retention.

The Assessment of the Musculoskeletal System

The muscles of the body are bilaterally assessed for size and symmetry. Contractures, tremors, weakness, paralysis, tremors, spasticity and/or flaccidity are identified and documented. The bones, and the areas around the bones, are assessed for any swelling, tenderness and deformities. All bodily joints are inspected for full range of motion, tenderness, and lesions.

The Assessment of the Neurological System

A complete neurological system assessment consists of:

- *Gross motor function and balance*

- *Fine motor function for both the upper and lower extremities*

- *Temperature sensation*

- *Kinesthetic sensation*

- *Sensory function*

- *Tactile sensation*

- *Cranial nerves*

- *Reflexes*

Gross Motor Function

There are several tools and methods that can be used to accomplish this task. The Romberg test is commonly used. This test involves having the patient stand with their arms to their sides while closing their eyes. Another alternative is to simply have the patient walk as you are monitoring their balance, coordination, gait, and gross motor movement. Having the patient stand on one foot with the eyes closed is a common test to assess the patient's balance. Toe-to-heel and heel-to-toe walking can be used to assess the patient's gait.

Fine Motor Function (FMF)

Higher extremity FMF is assessed by observing the patient's function and coordination in the hands and fingers; lower FMF is assessed by positioning the patient in supine, then asking them to place each of their heels on the opposite shin, as close to the knee as possible, and run them down their legs.

Temperature Sensation

Temperature sensation is assessed by touching various areas of the body, bilaterally, using warm and cool objects.

Kinesthetic Sensation

Kinesthetic sensation allows a person to perceive their bodily positioning without the use of any visual cues. This is assessed by moving the patient's fingers and toes in different directions while the patient's eyes are closed. The patient is then asked whether the digit is up, down or straight out as the assessor changes the positions without the help of visual cues.

Sensory Function

Using a pen, or another device, the assessor gently touches the surfaces of the body to determine whether or not the patient can feel it. The perception of pain is also assessed as part of sensory function. For this aspect, the assessor uses a both a sharp and a dull object to touch the patient's body and to determine if the patient can correctly identify the sensations.

Tactile Sensation

Tactile sensation and discrimination is the person's ability to perform the following while their eyes are closed:

- *One and two point discrimination.* During this phase of testing, the assessor touches the skin with either one or two pin pricks and the patient states how many pricks they feel.

- *Stereognosis.* A familiar item like a button, a pen, or a paper clip is placed in the person's hand with their eyes shut. The assessor then asks the person to identify the familiar object.

- *Extinction.* This test is performed by the assessor by simultaneously touching two symmetrical bodily areas, like both knees and both earlobes, and asking the patient if they feel one or two touches.

The Cranial Nerves

The twelve cranial nerves are:

- *Olfactory*
- *Optic*
- *Oculomotor*
- *Trochlear*
- *Trigeminal*
- *Abducens*
- *Facial*
- *Acoustic*
- *Glossopharyngeal*
- *Vagus*
- *Spinal accessory*
- *Hypoglossal*

Olfactory Nerve

This nerve is purely sensory. It transmits the sense of smell from the nasal cavity's olfactory foramina in the cribriform plate of the ethmoid bone.

Optic Nerve

This nerve is also purely sensory. It sends or transmits visual signals from the retina of the eye to the brain. This nerve is located in the optic canal.

Oculomotor Nerve

This nerve is primarily motor. It innervates various muscle groups which, in concert with each other, collectively perform most eye movements. It also innervates the ciliary bodies in the muscles and the sphincter papillae, which are located in the superior orbital fissure.

Trochlear Nerve

This motor nerve controls the superior oblique muscle. It is located in the superior aspect of the orbital fissure; it rotates and moves the eyeballs.

Trigeminal Nerve

This nerve is both motor and sensory. It receives stimulation from the face and innervates the muscles of mastication, or chewing muscles.

Abducens Nerve

This nerve is primarily motor, located in the superior orbital fissure. It innervates the lateral rectus which abducts the eye.

Facial Nerve

This nerve is both motor and sensory. This nerve originates in the internal acoustic canal. It innervates a variety of muscles that control facial expressions, the sense of taste from the anterior portion of the tongue, and provides secretomotor innervation to all of the salivary glands, with the exception of the parotid salivary gland and the lacrimal, or tear producing, glands.

Acoustic Nerve

This sensory nerve originates in the internal acoustic canal and senses gravity, sound, and rotation. It is necessary for bodily movement and balance. The vestibular branch carries impulses for equilibrium and the cochlear branch carries impulses for hearing.

Glossopharyngeal Nerve

This motor and sensory nerve, that is located in the jugular foramen, provides us with our sense of taste from the posterior aspect of the tongue. It provides secretomotor innervation to the parotid gland and motor signals to the stylopharyngeus (a muscle in the face and neck.)

Vagus Nerve

The vagus nerve is both motor and sensory and is located in the jugular foramen. The vagus nerve innervates the laryngeal and pharyngeal muscles; it also provides parasympathetic activity to virtually all of the abdominal and thoracic viscera and controls the resonance of the voice. Swallowing disorders like dysphasia originate from a disorder of this cranial nerve.

Spinal Accessory Nerve

The spinal accessory nerve is a motor nerve that innervates the trapezius and sternocleidomastoid muscles in concert with the vagus nerve. This cranial nerve is also anatomically located in the jugular foramen.

Hypoglossal Nerve

This motor nerve, located in the hypoglossal canal, is essential for swallowing and speech. It provides motor innervation to the tongue muscles with the exception of the palatoglossus muscle, which is innervated by other glossal muscles and the vagus cranial nerve.

Reflexes

A reflex is a muscle reaction that automatically occurs in response to a certain type of stimulus, or stimulation. Exaggerated, distorted, and absent reflexes can indicate serious nervous system pathology even before other abnormal neurological signs and symptoms appear. When reflexes are assessed, they must be assessed bilaterally in short succession so any differences can be noted. For example, when the assessors assesses the plantar reflex of the right limb, the same assessment should be done for the left limb immediately thereafter.

There are two types of reflexes. Some reflexes are present at the time of birth but they disappear shortly thereafter. Other reflexes are present at the time of birth and they remain active throughout the person's entire life. Some of the most common reflexes are the:

- *Plantar reflex*
- *Patellar tendon reflex*
- *Biceps reflex*
- *Calcaneal reflex*
- *Triceps reflex*
- *Pupil reflexes*

The plantar reflex involves plantar flexion of the foot. Normally, a stroke on the foot will cause the toes to move together and curl downward. An abnormal plantar reflex, referred to as the Babinski sign, occurs when the foot dorsiflexes, and the greater, or big toe, curls upward and the other toes flare out.

The assessor elicits the plantar reflex by drawing the handle of a Taylor hammer, or another blunt object, along the lateral side of the patient's sole, starting at the heel and ending on the ball of the foot near the big toe. A positive Babinski sign can indicate the presence of a life threatening disorder, such as deep vein thrombosis.

The biceps reflex is assessed by having the patient sit with their hands resting on their legs, and the assessor then places their thumb on the biceps tendon while simultaneously tapping the thumb with the Taylor hammer. Similarly, the triceps reflex is elicited bilaterally by having the patient sit with their hands resting on their legs as the assessor lightly holds the patient's forearm when simultaneously tapping the triceps tendon, which is located just above the elbow.

The patellar tendon reflex, often referred to as the knee-jerk reflex, is assessed by sharply tapping or striking the patellar. The calcaneal reflex, also referred to as the ankle-jerk reflex and the Achilles reflex, is elicitedby sharply tapping the calcaneal tendon ankle with the base of a Taylor hammer.

Pupil reflexes include pupil dilation and accommodation. The mnemonic "PERLA" is useful for the assessment. PERLA stands for Pupils Equally Reactive to Light and Accommodation. Pupil dilation is assessed in a dimly lit room. Place the edge of your hand on the bridge of the patient's nose to separate each eye and its field of vision. Then bring a flashlight from the side of the face to within 5 to 10 cm of the subject's face while shining the light into each eye to assess and determine the pupils' responses to light. Did the pupils normally constrict with the light? Did the pupils constrict equally and identically for both eyes? Asking the patient to look into the distance and then look at an object close to their face is done to assess pupillary accommodation. The pupils normally constrict when an object is close to their face; and the pupils should normally dilate when an object is farther away. Do the pupils constrict and dilate, as they should? Are the responses the same for both eyes?

Other reflexes present at birth and throughout life include:

- *Gag Reflex:* When the throat or back of the mouth is stimulated, causing gagging

- *Sneeze Reflex:* Sneezing from irritation in the nasal passages

- *Blinking Reflex:* Blinking eyes when they are touched or a bright light suddenly appears

- *Cough Reflex:* Coughing from stimulation in the airway

- *Yawn Reflex:* Yawning when the body needs more oxygen

Infant Reflexes

Infant reflexes, also referred to as primitive reflexes, are a highly important sign of nervous system development and function. If these primitive reflexes remain past the expected age of disappearance, it can be a sign of damage to the brain or nervous system.

Primitive Reflexes	Description
Sucking Reflex	This reflex is linked to the rooting reflex. The infant instinctively sucks anytime something, like a finger or a nipple, touches the area around the mouth or on the roof of the mouth.
Rooting Reflex	The infant will turn toward the side that is stroked and makes sucking motions.
Moro (Startle) Reflex	The Moro, or startle reflex, is elicited with sudden noises and other sudden changes like environmental temperature occur. The legs and head extend while the arms move up and out with the palms facing upwards and thumbs flexed. Then the arms come together, with the hands clenching into fists, and the infant cries. This reflex typically disappears at around 3 or 4 months of age.
Step Reflex	When the soles of the infant's feet touch a flat surface they will try to "walk" by putting one foot in front of the other. The step or walking reflex also begins at birth and it disappears at about six to eight weeks of age.
Tonic Neck Reflex	Tonic neck reflex happens when you move a child's to the side and the arm on the same side of where the head faces reaches away from the body with the hand partially open. The arm on the opposite side flexes with the

	fist tightly clenched. If the baby's face is turned in the opposite direction, the position is reversed. The tonic neck position is sometimes called the fencer's position since it resembles a fencer's stance.
The Galant (Truncal Incurvation) Reflex	The Galant, or truncal incurvation reflex, happens when the infant is stroked or tapped along the side of the spine when the infant lies on their stomach, resulting in the infant twitching his or her hips toward the touch.
The Grasp Reflex	Newborns have strong grasps and the grasp reflex occurs when you place a finger on the infant's open palm, resulting in the hand closing around the finger. Trying to remove the finger results in the infant tightening their grip.

The Assessment of the Male and Female Genitalia and Lymph Nodes

For both genders, the assessor inspects the inguinal lymph nodes and the pubis for swelling, infection, inflammation and/or infestation, and they assess the pubic hair for characteristics, amount, and distribution.

For the male, the assessor also assesses the penis, urethral meatus, and the scrotum for swelling, signs of inflammation, tenderness, and any discharge. For the female, the assessor separates the labia, examines the skin, the clitoris, the vagina, and the urethral opening.

The Assessment of the Rectum and Anus

The anal sphincter is palpated to determine tone, masses, tenderness, or nodules with a finger of a gloved hand. The glove is then examined for any signs of obvious blood.

NEONATAL AND PEDIATRIC MODIFICATIONS AND IMPLICATIONS

In addition to the variations in terms of physical assessment and the implications of findings addressed above, some other variations for neonates and other members of the pediatric population, as listed below, will be discussed here.

- *Respiratory rate and regularity*
- *Blood Pressure*
- *Pulses*
- *Arterial blood gases*
- *Posture*
- *Skin*
- *Head*
- *Eyes, ears, nose and mouth*

- *Sensory functioning*
- *Neck*
- *Chest*
- *Abdomen*
- *Anogenital area*
- *Extremities*
- *Spine*
- *Reflexes*

Respiratory Rate and Regularity

All neonates have irregular breathing patterns. For example, they may breathe at the rate of 80 breaths per minute after which they have a slower rate for a brief period of time. Premature infants often have periodic breathing which is a pattern of intermittent apnea lasting up to five seconds; in contrast, apnea is defined as the cessation or pause in breathing for long than 20 seconds. Apnea is an abnormal respiratory assessment that must be thoroughly assessed and explored in order to determine its etiology. Apnea can be accompanied with cyanosis, pallor, hypotonic muscles, and bradycardia.

Neonates are also assessed for the signs of respiratory distress using the Silverman scoring system. This scoring system rates the neonate's respiratory distress according to a Grade 0, Grade 1, or Grade 2 for each of the following assessments:

- Upper chest movement
- Lower chest movement
- Xiphoid retraction
- Dilation of the nares
- Expiratory grunting

The signs of respiratory distress include nasal flaring during inspiration, grunting as the result of an effort to increase the end expiratory pressure, and xiphoid as well as chest wall retractions at the intercostal, subcostal, substernal, and suprasternal areas which indicates an obstructed airway or diminished lung compliance. Although chest wall retractions can occur among all ages, it is most pronounced and dramatic among neonates because the chest cage is not yet rigid, and is thinner and weaker than those of older children and adults.

Some common neonatal respiratory disorders are:

- *IRDS*
    - *Tachypnea, refractions, grunting , nasal flaring, cyanosis, diminished breath sounds, and rales*

- *Pneumothorax*
    - *Tachypnea, refractions, grunting , nasal flaring, cyanosis, diminished breath sounds and asymmetrical chest movement*

- *Pneumonia*
    - *Apnea, tachypnea, refractions, grunting , nasal flaring, cyanosis, rales and rhonchi*

- *Upper Airway Obstruction*
    - *Apnea, tachypnea, grunting, stridor, labored breathing and gasping.*

- *Diaphragmatic Hernia*

  o *Tachypnea, grunting, nasal flaring, cyanosis, and bowel sounds in the chest*

- *Meconium Aspiration*

  o *Apnea, tachypnea, refractions, grunting, nasal flaring, stridor, cyanosis, and diminished breath sounds*

- *Transient Tachypnea*

  o *Tachypnea, refractions, grunting , nasal flaring, and fine rales*

- *Apnea of Prematurity*

  o *Apnea, refractions, nasal flaring, and cyanosis*

Normal breath sounds among the pediatric population have longer and louder inspirations when compared to expirations.

Blood Pressure

Blood pressures for smaller birth weight neonates are lower than those listed in the table above. For example, a neonate weighing 600g may have a blood pressure of 45/20 and a mean blood pressure of 25mm Hg, and a neonate between 1,000 and 2,000g may have a blood pressure of 48/25 and a mean blood pressure of 35 mm Hg. The calculation of the adequate mean blood pressure for gestational age in weeks is gestational age in weeks + 5

Pulses

Weak pulses many indicate the presence of hypo-plastic left-sided heart syndrome, shock, and other causes of low cardiac output; bounding pulses can indicate left to right shunting and a patent ductus arteriosus, and this is typically accompanied with a widened pulse pressure and decreases in the systolic blood pressure. Under normal circumstances, the upper extremity blood pressures should be higher than those of the lower extremities, and the brachial and femoral pulses should have equal intensity.

Arterial Blood Gases

An arterial blood gas analysis provides information on oxygenation of blood through gas exchange in the patient's lungs, carbon dioxide (CO_2) elimination through respiration, and acid-base balance or imbalance in the patient's extra-cellular fluid (ECF).

Parameter	Normal Range
pH	7.35-7.45
PaCO2	35-45
PaO2	80-100
HCO3 (bicarbonate)	22-26 mEq/L
BE (base excess)	-2 +/- 2
SO2 (calculated via PO2, as above)	95-100%

The normal values for premature infants (according to gestational age) and for infants and children up to two years of age is below:

Arterial Blood Gas	Premature Infant < 28 Weeks	Premature Infant < 40 Weeks	Infants and Children < 2 Years
pH	7.25	7.25	7.3 to 7.4
Paco2	45 to 55	45 to 55	30 to 40
Pao2	45 to 65	50 to 70	80 to 100
Bicarbonate	15 to 18	18 to 20	20 to 22

When interpreting primary acid-base disturbances, evaluate acid-base status before oxygenation. The pH and $PaCO_2$ are considered in order to determine the basic acid-base status. Determining whether the pH is normal (7.35-7.45), low (<7.35 "acidemia"), or high (>7.45 "alkalemia"), is the first step. Next the $PaCO_2$ is assessed, and if the pH is normal and the $PaCO_2$ is also normal, then the acid-base balance is normal. If the pH is low, the primary disturbance must be either respiratory acidosis (high $PaCO_2$) or metabolic acidosis (low $PaCO_2$); when the pH is high, it indicates that the primary disturbance must be either respiratory alkalosis ($PaCO_2$ < 35 torr) or metabolic alkalosis ($PaCO_2$ > 35 torr.)

Basic arterial blood gas interpretation requires that the different categories of hypoxemia are also recognized. The categories are as follows:

- *Mild: 60-79 torr*
- *Moderate: 40-59 torr*
- *Severe < 40 torr*

Underlying Disorder	Typical ABG Result	Interpretation
Moderate to severe COPD with CO2 retention	pH = 7.36 PaCO2 = 58 torr PaO2 = 62 torr HCO3 = 30 mEq/L BE +- 7	Fully compensated respiratory acidosis with mild hypoxemia
Pneumonia, pulmonary emboli, or any other condition associated with moderate to severe hypoxemia	pH 7.52 PaCO2 27 torr PaO2 48 torr HCO3 22mEq/L BE-1	Uncompensated respiratory alkalosis with moderate hypoxemia. The alkalosis may be a result of tachypnea associated with hypoxemia.

Posture

Under normal circumstances, the neonate resists the extension of the extremities and lies in a fetal position with the arms and legs flexed.

Skin

The skin should have no signs of jaundice or cyanosis, and the texture is soft, smooth, and dry. Some irregularities include vernix caseosa, a thick cheesy skin covering; fine hair, referred to as lanugo; milia, which are small raised spots, and can be white or red; telangiectatic nevi, also referred to as stork bites; Mongolian spots, which are purple-blue in color; nevus flammeus, or a port wine stain; and erythema neonatorum, or erythema toxicum, which is a pink rash. These findings do not indicate neonatal abnormalities, and most disappear in a couple of days or weeks, with the exception of nevus flammeus, which can be permanent and distressing to the parents.

Head

Normally, the head's circumference is 2-3 cm greater than the neonate's chest circumference. Measurements greater than this can indicate hydrocephalus; measurements less than this can indicate microcephaly.

The fontanels should be flat and soft with occasional minor bulging during crying. Other bulging can indicate neonatal infection, hemorrhage, or increased intracranial pressure; dehydration is signaled with depressed fontanels.

The sutures should be separated, and there is often some normal molding as the result of the birth process. Caput succedaneum, swelling of the neonate's scalp, and cephalohematomas can be temporarily present under normal circumstances as the result of birth trauma and the pressure exerted on the head during labor and delivery.

Eyes, Ears, Nose and Mouth

The normal neonatal eyes are equal in terms of shape and size, and normally spaced, with the exception of Down syndrome. The red and the papillary reflexes are present, appearing blue or gray with changes over the next year; movement is jerky and not smooth and coordinated, and there may be some small hemorrhages in the conjunctivae from birth trauma.

The ears should be normally placed, the cartilage should be well formed and firm to the touch, there should be no skin tags, and the neonate should respond to noises and voices. Low-set ears can signal Down syndrome or a renal disorder; a lack of ear cartilage can signal prematurity.

The nose is normally midline, without a bridge, and without drainage other than some mucus. Neonates are nasal breathers and they are able to sneeze.

Normally, the mouth has a closed palate, symmetrical lip movements, Epstein pearls (small white oral cysts that disappear spontaneously) a symmetrical, non-protruding tongue, pink oral mucosa without signs of fungal infection like Candida albicans, and little saliva. Excessive saliva can indicate tracheoesophageal fistula; a protruding tongue is a sign of Down syndrome.

Sensory Functioning

As previously stated, the neonate should normally respond to sounds. Additionally, the neonate should also be able to sense tactile stimuli (touch), gustatory stimuli (taste) like sour and bitter, and visual stimuli like light and objects about 12 inches from the face.

Neck

The neck should freely move up and down and from side to side with a minimal amount of control. A complete lack of control can indicate Down syndrome and/or prematurity.

Chest

The breast nodule should be 6 mm and the nipples should be well-formed, bilaterally symmetrical, and without any visible defects. The shape is round and barrel-like and without any retractions. Respirations are diaphragmatic and the clavicles should be intact without signs of birth trauma.

Abdomen

The normal neonatal abdomen is round and not distended; bowel sounds should be present within a couple of hours after birth, and the umbilical cord and umbilical site should be odorless and free of any signs of infection, respectively.

Anogenital Area

Normally, the neonate passes meconium about 24 hours or less after birth, the testes are in the scrotum, the male has scrotal rugae, and the urinary meatus is on the tip of the penis. The female neonate may have some edema of the labia, the labia majora should cover the clitoris and the labia minora, and the hymen should be present. At times, maternal pregnancy hormones may cause the neonate's vagina to bleed lightly, but this is of no concern.

All neonates should produce urine in less than 24 hours; the color may be rusty in color for a couple of days as the result of the presence of uric acid crystals. The anus should be open and not covered with any membranes.

Extremities

Normal extremities have symmetrical full range of motion. They are normally flexed and capable of spontaneous movement. Additionally, the gluteal folds should be symmetrical, no hip abduction click should be heard, and the extremity nail beds should be pink.

Spine

Under normal circumstances, the spine should be midline, flat, straight, easily flexed, and without any openings, as can occur with spina bifida.

LABORATORY DATA

Respiratory therapists review and interpret the results of a number of laboratory tests including:

- *A complete blood count*
- *Coagulation studies*

Complete Blood Count (CBC)

A complete blood count (CBC) determines the number of white blood cells (WBC), the number of red blood cells (RBC), the platelet count, the portion of the blood that contains red blood cells which is referred to as the hematocrit, and the total amount of hemoglobin in the blood.

A complete blood count (CBC) is used to diagnose and monitor a wide variety of health disorders including anemia, infection, inflammation, leukemia, bleeding disorders, clotting disorders as well as abnormal blood cell destruction and production.

White Blood Cells

In addition to the white blood cell count (WBC), a CBC can also measure the white blood cell differential which counts the number of each of the five types of white blood cells in the blood, (namely, the lymphocytes, neutrophils, monocytes, basophils, and eosinophils), and determine the number of band cells, which are immature neutrophils, T-type lymphocytes or T cells, and B-type lymphocytes or B cells.

Leukopenia, or an abnormally low WBC count, can occur as the result of impaired bone marrow functioning, an autoimmune disease such as systemic lupus erythematous, hepatic disease, viral infections, and a disorder of the spleen. Patients with leukopenia, regardless of cause, are at greater risk for infection than other patients with a normal WBC count.

Leukocytosis, or an elevated WBC count, can result from inflammatory diseases such as arthritis, infections such as tuberculosis and pneumonia, sepsis, leukemia, physical and emotional stress, and extensive tissue damage such as that which occurs as the result of a burn.

The normal white blood count is 4,500 to 10,000 cells/mcL.

Red Blood Cells

Other things that the CBC measures and determines is the amount of oxygen-carrying hemoglobin in each red blood cell (RBC), which is referred to as the MCH or the mean corpuscular hemoglobin; the amount or concentration of hemoglobin in relation to the size of the RBC, which is referred to as MCHC or mean corpuscular hemoglobin concentration; the average size of the red blood cells, which is referred to as the MCV or mean corpuscular volume; red cell distribution width (RDW) which measures the variations of the sizes of the red blood cells; and the reticulocyte count which reflects the number or percentage of immature, young blood cells.

Elevated RBC counts and hematocrit can occur from a variety of causes such as smoking, dehydration, renal disease, lung disease, and polycythemia vera. Polycythemia is defined as an excessive red blood cell count and secondary polycythemia is defined as an excessive red blood cell count that results from chronic hypoxemia as can occur with a congenial heart disorder and chronic obstructive pulmonary disease and other pulmonary or cardiac disorders. Patients with polycythemia are at risk for blood clotting and increased after load because the blood is thickened in the presence of polycythemia.

Low RBCs and hematocrit can result from anemia, hemorrhage, chronic renal disease, infections such as hepatitis, impaired bone marrow function as can occur secondary to radiation therapy, leukemia, multiple myeloma, some autoimmune disorders such as rheumatoid arthritis, red blood cell destruction which is referred to as hemolysis and inadequate nutrition that is lacking in iron, folate, vitamin B12 and/or vitamin B6.

Low hemoglobin can be secondary to hemorrhage and all types of anemia.

The normal red blood count for males is 4.7 to 6.1 million cells/mcL and, for females, the normal red blood count is 4.2 to 5.4 million cells/mcL.

The normal hematocrit for males is 40.7 to 50.3% and, for females, the normal hematocrit is 36.1 to 44.3%; the normal hemoglobin for males is 13.8 to 17.2 gm/dL and the normal hemoglobin for females is

12.1 to 15.1 gm/dL. Other normal values related to the red blood cells include:

- *MCH: 27 to 31 pg/cell*
- *MCHC: 32 to 36 gm/dL*
- *MCV: 80 to 95 femtoliter*

Coagulation Studies

Coagulation studies can include direct measures such as those that measure the number of platelets, also referred to as thrombocytes, and indirect measures to see how effectively, or ineffectively, the platelets are functioning. These indirect measures are referred to as platelet function assays.

Platelets coagulate the blood and prevent bleeding by clumping together with other platelets, sticking to the site of the bleeding, and by releasing substances that stimulate aggregation. They are produced by the bone marrow.

Some assays that measure platelet function are:

- *Closure time assays*

This test measures the closure time for the platelets to coagulate when exposed to an activating substance.

- *Thromboelastometry or Viscoelastometry*

This test measures the strength of the blood clot has it is formed.

- *Endpoint Bead or Endpoint Platelet Aggregation Assay*

This test measures the number of platelets that collect and aggregate after an activating substance is added to the blood sample.

- *Bleeding Time*

This direct measurement of platelet functioning, although not done as often as it was in the past, reflects the amount of time that it takes for bleeding to stop.

- *Platelet Aggregometry*

Platelet aggregometry consists of a number of different tests, all of which measure the aggregation of the platelets after an activating substance has been added to the sample.

- *Flow Cytometry*

Flow cytometry uses lasers to detect proteins on the surface of the platelet and how these proteins change when an activating agent is added.

Patients with excessive and fast clotting are at risk for the formation of blood clots and emboli; patients with a slow or impaired clotting response are at risk for bleeding, therefore, all venipuncture and arterial puncture sites must have pressure applied to them to prevent bleeding.

Sputum Testing and Gram Staining

Some bacteria are classified as gram positive because they react to a Gram stain; these microbes have thick walls containing teichoic acid and peptidoglycan. Others are classified as gram negative because they do not react to a Gram stain. These microbes, more common than gram positive bacteria, have thinner walls than gram positive bacteria; these walls are comprised of peptidoglycan and a lipid membrane which includes lipoproteins and lipopolysaccharides, which are endotoxins.

Some examples of gram positive bacteria include streptococcus pneumonia (pneumococci), staphylococci which can lead to respiratory and cardiac infections such as endocarditis and pneumonia, and streptococci which can cause pneumonia, bronchitis, pharyngitis, rheumatic fever, and endocarditis.

Examples of gram positive bacteria associated with respiratory diseases include haemophilus influenzae, legionella pneumophilia, and yersinia pseudotuberculosis.

Bacteria are also differentiated by their ability to resist color changes when subjected to a staining procedure in the laboratory. Acid fast bacteria resist decolorization when stained with a Ziehl-Neelsen or Kinyoun stain, for example.

Sputum specimens, including sputum cultures, are normally without any pathogenic organisms. When the sputum is cultured and the findings are abnormal, it can be an indication of a number of disorders and diseases such as a bacterial, viral or fungal infection, bronchitis, cystic fibrosis, chronic obstructive pulmonary disease, a lung abscess, pneumonia, and tuberculosis.

Electrolytes

Electrolyte panels, alone or in combination with a metabolic panel, are used to both diagnose disorders and to monitor the outcomes of care for a particular disorder that can, or does, impact on the fluid, electrolyte, and acid base balances of the body. For example, a patient with edema will have an electrolyte panel to diagnose their disorder, and a patient with chronic heart failure needs electrolyte panels to monitor this chronic disorder.

Electrolytes and fluids are transported through the body with both active and passive transport processes. Passive transport processes include diffusion, osmosis, and filtration. The process of diffusion moves fluids and electrolytes from an area of higher concentration to an area of lower concentration; osmosis moves fluids through a selectively permeable membrane in the presence of at least one impermeable solute; and filtration moves fluids and small solute particles through a filtration membrane from an area of high pressure to area of low pressure. Active transport moves molecules across cell membranes from an area of lower concentration to an area of higher concentration as occurs with the movement of glucose and amino acids.

Electrolytes are ions that can have either a negative or positive charge when the number of electrons is either greater than or less than the number of protons. Cations have a positive charge, and anions have a negative charge.

The cations are:

- *Sodium (Na+)*
- *Potassium (K+)*
- *Calcium (Ca+)*
- *Magnesium (Mg++)*

The anions include:

- *Chloride (Cl-)*

- *Bicarbonate (HCO3-)*

- *Sulfate (SO4-)*

- *Hydrogen phosphate (HPO4-)*

Although excesses and deficits of each of the electrolytes have specific signs and symptoms, the general symptoms that may occur with an electrolyte imbalance include fatigue, nausea without vomiting, dizziness, trembling, constipation, dark urine, decreased urine output, muscle weakness, stiff or aching joints, dry skin, dry mouth, and bad breath. Serious symptoms are poor elasticity of the skin, tachycardia, sunken eyes, and a change in mental status, such as confusion, delirium, hallucinations, or delusions. The normal levels for some electrolytes and glucose are:

- *Potassium:* 3.5 to 5.5 mEq/L

- *Sodium:* 135 to 145 mEq/L

- *Chloride*: 95 to 106 mEq/L

- *Bicarbonate:* 22 to 25 mEq/L

- *Calcium:* 4.5 to 5.5 mEq/L

- *Glucose:* 60 to 110 mg/100 mL

Electrolyte	Excesses	Deficiencies
Potassium	Hyperkalemia: Cardiac changes such as high T waves, widened QRS complex, depressed ST segment, bradycardia, and flaccid paralysis	Hypokalemia: Cardiac changes such as depressed ST segment, inverted or flat T waves, premature ventricular contractions, ventricular fibrillation and cardiac arrest if left untreated, and muscular weakness
Sodium	Hypernatremia: The signs and symptoms of dehydration	Hyponatremia: Fluid overload

Chloride	Hyperchloremia: The prolongation of the QT interval and the ST segment	Hypochloremia: A wider or more rounded T wave and a shortened QT interval
Bicarbonate	Bicarbonate retention to compensate for respiratory acidosis that occurs as the result of an elevated carbon dioxide level	The excessive excretion of bicarbonate to compensate for respiratory alkalosis that occurs as the result of a decreased carbon dioxide level
Glucose	Hyperglycemia Fatigue, blurred vision, excessive thirst, headache, frequent urination, hyperosmolar syndrome, ketoacidosis, and long term complications such as renal failure, nephropathy, and diabetic retinopathy This is most typically the result of the poor	Hypoglycemia Excessive hunger, sweating, anxiety, shakiness, heart palpitations, double or blurry vision, confusion, loss of consciousness, seizures, coma, and death This is associated with diabetics who have taken too much insulin, too little food, or have exercised excessively.

management of diabetes.

The treatment of electrolyte imbalances is dependent on what type of electrolyte is actually affected. For example, a patient with low potassium levels should be urged to eat high potassium foods, to take potassium supplements, and they may be given intravenous supplementation. If a patient's potassium levels are high, the patient may be treated with diuretics.

In addition to the immediate treatment for electrolyte imbalances, it is vital that the cause for the imbalance is discovered and corrected. Possible causes include kidney disease, hormone/endocrine problems, stomach disorders, an improper diet, a loss of bodily fluids due to illness, and as the result of side effects of chemotherapy or medications.

Some types of medications that can cause an electrolyte imbalance in the body are steroids, tricyclic antidepressants, birth control pills, diuretics, cough medicines, laxatives, steroids, and excessive use of antacids.

Cultures and Sensitivity Testing

When a culture and sensitivity is indicated, as based on the patient's clinical condition, the sample is microscopically examined, after which it is cultured in an appropriate medium such as a nutrient broth or agar. Cultures are useful for the identification of the microorganism, to determine whether the wound, for example, is colonized or infected and also to get a numeric values for the colony.

Sensitivity testing entails subjecting the culture to a number of different antibiotics in order to confirm whether or not the pathogen is treatable and sensitive to specific antibiotics or if it is resistant to the antibiotic, as is the case with methicillin-resistant Staphylococcus aureus (MRSA.)

Specimens for microbiology, culture, and sensitivity must be collected correctly and processed as soon as possible after collection because some microorganisms may not survive prolonged lengths of time before the laboratory processes them.

The use of antimicrobials for the treatment of infections is the most common therapeutic treatment. To the greatest extent possible, the selection of the antimicrobial and the dosage should be driven by the specific microorganism and the current physical condition of the host.

Antimicrobial prophylaxis can be a primary prevention or a secondary prevention measure. It is considered primary prevention when it prevents any infection, and it is considered secondary prevention when it treats and prevents the recurrence of an infection.

Antimicrobial prophylaxis is often, and perhaps too often, used to prevent the onset of an infectious disease. For example, preventive prophylactic antibiotics can be used for the prevention of urinary tract infections when a patient has an indwelling urinary catheter, and to prevent other infections such as rheumatic fever which can lead to serious cardiac damage, herpes simplex, recurring bouts of cellulitis, meningitis, endocarditis, as well as open wounds and open fracture infections.

Prophylactic antimicrobials, particularly antibiotics, are also used, and indicated, perioperatively for certain types of surgery, like gastrointestinal and total joint replacement surgical procedures, to prevent surgically related infections. For example, an intravenous antibiotic may be administered ½ hour to 1 hour prior to a surgical procedure.

Ideally, prophylactic antimicrobials should not be used, however, when it is necessary to use them they must be used judiciously. The ideal prophylactic antimicrobial should be limited in terms of the duration of use, inexpensive, nontoxic, target specific and bactericidal. Resistance remains a high public health concern.

The therapeutic use of antimicrobials should, under ideal circumstances be based on the components of the cycle of infection. For example, it should be based on the site of the infection, the host, and whenever possible, based on a definitive diagnosis of the infection and the offending pathogen. At times, when there is not yet a definitive diagnosis, the empiric use of antimicrobials is indicated.

The identification of the specific offending pathogen is extremely important especially when an infection can be life threatening, when the patient is not responding to current therapeutic interventions, and when the course of antimicrobial therapy is anticipated to be rather prolonged.

This accurate identification is dependent upon accurate and timely microbiological laboratory testing prior to the initiation of the therapy, whenever possible. In addition to laboratory testing, the patient's past medical history, including an exposure history, and the presenting signs and symptoms also serve as considerations in terms of exactly which antimicrobial is the most effective and the most appropriate for the patient.

The initiation of the antimicrobial therapy is based on a number of considerations including the condition of the patient. For example, critically ill patients, like those with sepsis, should have an initiation of antimicrobial therapy immediately after diagnostic specimens are obtained. When the patient condition is stable, it is recommended that antimicrobial therapy be postponed until laboratory findings are complete.

The empiric use of antimicrobials is defined as the use of antimicrobial medications based on empiric signs and symptoms in the patient's physical condition because microbiological results typically do not get done in less than 24 to 72 hours.

The antimicrobial agents that are used with empiric, rather than definitive, diagnoses are typically broad scope agents or a combination of agents until a definitive diagnosis is done.

Other Laboratory Tests for Infections

Other commonly used blood laboratory tests used for infections includes the erythrocyte sedimentation rate (ESR), C-reactive protein (CRP), and plasma viscosity (PV), all of which are sensitive to the increases in protein, which is a part of the inflammation process. The ESR, CRP, and PV can be raised with primarily bacterial infections, abscesses, and other disorders such as cancer, burns, and a myocardial infarction. Some health problems like polycythemia, sickle cell anemia, and heart failure can be signaled with a less than normal ESR. Additionally, urine testing and spinal fluid analysis can also be done.

- *The Erythrocyte Sedimentation Rate (ESR)*

The erythrocyte sedimentation rate (ESR) measures the rate with which the red blood cells separate from the plasma and fall to the bottom of the test tube within a given period of time. A high erythrocyte sedimentation rate indicates the presence of infection because the proteins of infection cover the red blood cells thus causing them to fall more rapidly.

The normal erythrocyte sedimentation rate (ESR) for females is 0-20 millimeters per hour and the normal rate for males is 0-15 millimeters per hour. The normal sedimentation rate among elders can be slightly higher.

- *C Reactive Protein*

  C reactive protein, sometimes referred to as the acute phase of inflammation protein, can rise as high as 1000 times normal when infection and inflammation occur. It can also rise with burns, surgery, and cancer.

  The normal C reactive protein is < 1.0 mg/dL or less than 10 mg/L

- *Plasma Viscosity*

  Simply stated, blood viscosity is the thickness of the blood. Some of the factors that impact on the viscosity of blood include plasma viscosity, or thickness, the hematocrit, the level of red blood cell aggregation, and temperature. Higher temperatures lead to lower viscosity and lower temperatures lead to increase blood thickness and viscosity.

  The normal viscosity of the blood, at 37 °C, is 3×10^{-3} to 4×10^{-3}.

- *Urine Tests*

  More than 100 different tests can be done on urine. A regular, or routine, urinalysis includes the color, clarity, odor, specific gravity, pH, proteins, glucose, ketones, nitrites, leukocyte esterase, and microscopic evaluation.

  Bacteria can make normally clear urine cloudy. Infections can also make urine odorous. In the presence of a urinary tract infection, nitrites will be present and the leukocyte esterase will show white blood cells, or leukocytes in the urine.

  Microscopic analysis is done after the urine is centrifuged to render sediment for analysis. Some of the things that can be found in urine with microscopic analysis include the abnormal presence of red and/or white blood cells which indicates inflammation and infection, casts which can also indicate infection, crystals in the presence of stones, and bacteria, yeast, and/or parasites when an infection is present.

- *Spinal Taps*

  Spinal taps, also referred to as a lumbar puncture, is also done to determine if the cerebrospinal fluid is infected, as is the case with meningitis. Normal values for ccrebrospinal fluids are:

  - *A pressure of 70 - 180 mm H20*

  - *A colorless and clear appearance*

  - *15 - 60 mg/100 mL of total protein*

  - *3 - 12% of the total protein is gamma globulin*

  - *50 - 80 mg/100 mL glucose*

  - *0 - 5 mononuclear white blood cells*

  - *No red blood cells*

  - *110 - 125 mEq/L chloride*

Increased CSF pressure occurs as the result of increased intracranial pressure secondary to a head injury, for example. Protein can increase with an infection or any other inflammatory process; glucose can be decreased with infections like meningitis and tuberculosis; increased white blood cells can indicate an acute infection; and red blood cells indicate bleeding.

IMAGING STUDIES

Diagnostic imaging tests are used to assess pulmonary disorders and to determine the morbidity and mortality of the affected patients:

- *X-rays*

- *Cardiac catheterization and angiography*

- *12 lead ECG*

- *Echocardiography*

- *Fluoroscopy*

- *Computed tomography*

- *CT angiography*

- *MRI*

- *Nuclear scanning*

- *Ultrasonography*

X-rays

X-rays that are used to image the chest and assess pulmonary status include a simple x-ray, fluoroscopy, CT angiography, and high resolution and spiral or helical CT. The most common imaging study for the majority of pulmonary patients is a simple chest x-ray.

Plain chest x-rays and fluoroscopy images the lungs and surrounding structures. Plain chest x-rays images, most often the initial imaging study, allow the identification and diagnosis of a number of abnormalities including those related to the hilum, the mediastinum, the pleura, the chest wall, the diaphragm, the lung parenchyma, and the heart.

Standard chest x-rays can be done with a lateral, anterior posterior, a lateral decubitus, lordotic or apical lordotic, and an oblique view. The oblique view is useful to assess the pulmonary nodules and to rule out abnormalities that occur because of superimposed structural images. The lateral view, although not as effective as a CT, provides data relating to pleural effusion; and an end expiratory x-ray can provide information about small pneumothoraxes. Lastly, a screening chest x-ray is done when a patient has a positive tuberculin skin test without any symptoms.

Cardiac Catheterization and Angiography

Cardiac catheterization is a diagnostic procedure that entails the passing of a catheter into the pulmonary artery, the coronary artery, the chambers of the heart, the coronary vein, or the pulmonary vein.

This procedure can perform a variety of cardiac tests including cardiac output measurement, myocardial metabolism measurements, and the measurement of cardiac functioning; it is also used to visualize the anatomy of the heart and the coronary artery. Angiography, shunt detection, and intravascular ultrasonography can also be done with cardiac catheterization.

Cardiac cauterizations include left and right heart catheterizations. Left heart catheterization is performed with a subclavian, femoral, brachial or radial artery entry and it is helpful for the assessment of the coronary artery anatomy, aortic valve function, mitral valve function, systemic vascular resistance, left ventricular function, and pressure and the aortic blood pressure.

Right heart catheterization is performed with the catheter passing into the right atrium, the tricuspid valve, and then into the right ventricle across the pulmonary valve and then into the pulmonary artery. The possible catheter entry sites include the jugular, femoral, subclavian, and antecubital veins. Right heart catheterization is helpful for the assessments of pulmonary artery occlusion pressure, pulmonic valve functioning, tricuspid valve functioning, right atrial pressure, right ventricular pressure, pulmonary vascular resistance, and pulmonary artery pressure. These assessments are often beneficial to the diagnosis of pericarditis, cardiac tamponade, and cardiomyopathy.

A number of different cardiac tests and diagnostic procedures can be performed during cardiac catheterization including:

- *Angiography*

- *Intravascular ultrasonography*

- *The measurement of cardiac output (CO)*

- *The detection and exploration any cardiac anatomical anomalies*

- *An endomyocardial biopsy*

- *Measurements of myocardial metabolism*

12 Lead ECG

A standard 12 lead ECG provides us with the electrical activity of the heart with 12 different vector views.

An ECG machine uses standardized graph paper with time, or duration, on the x axis and voltage on the y axis. Each square on the graph paper is 1 millimeter and bolder divisions on the graph paper are 5 millimeters.

A typical ECG is comprised of a P wave, a QRS complex, a T wave, and a U wave, which is often not detectable because it is hidden with the T wave or the next P wave.

The P wave is the depolarization or activation of the atria. The QRS complex is the ventricular depolarization and it is typically from 0.07 to 0.10 seconds. When this interval is from 0.10 to 0.11 seconds, indicates incomplete bundle branch block or an intra-ventricular conduction delay and when it is 0.12 seconds or more, it indicates complete bundle branch block or an intra-ventricular conduction delay. The T wave is ventricular repolarization and the U wave is the relaxation of the ventricles after depolarization. The T wave is usually rounded and smooth; hypo-magnesemia and hypokalemia are signaled when the amplitude or height of the T wave is low and left ventricular hypertrophy; hyperkalemia and hypo-calcemia are signaled when the T wave is peaked and high.

The PR interval is the amount of time that elapses between the beginning of atrial depolarization until the onset of ventricular and normally it is from 0.10 seconds and 0.20 seconds; when the PR interval is prolonged, it indicates 1st degree atrioventricular block. The QT interval is the amount of time that elapses between the onset of ventricular depolarization and the end of ventricular repolarization. The R-R interval is the duration of time between two successive QRS complexes.

Lastly, the ST segment reflects complete ventricular depolarization and when the ST segment is abnormally depressed, it can indicate hypokalemia or an acute myocardial infarction and when the ST segment is abnormally elevated, it suggests a number of different abnormalities such as:

- *Hypothermia*
- *A pulmonary embolism*
- *Left ventricular aneurysm*
- *Left ventricular hypertrophy*

- *Myocardial ischemia*
- *Myocardial infarction*
- *Pericarditis*
- *Hyperkalemia*

Although the U wave can be present in patients without any abnormality, it can also occur when the patient is affected with ischemia, hypomagnesaemia, and hypokalemia.

Echocardiography

Echocardiography images the great vessels of the heart and the heart itself. This diagnostic test is beneficial for determining the thickness of the heart wall in terms of hypertrophy and atrophy, diastolic filling of the left ventricle, the presence of cardiomyopathy, pulmonary emboli, aortic regurgitation, heart failure, and areas of infarction or ischemia.

Echocardiograms can be done with the transthoracic, the most commonly used technique, or the transesophageal method. They can be performed in two dimensions and three dimensions, the latter of which is particularly useful for assessing the mitral valve.

The types of echocardiography are:

- *Contrast echocardiography*

- *Spectral Doppler echo-cardiography*

- *Color Doppler echo-cardiography*

- *Tissue Doppler imaging*

- *Three-dimensional echocardiography*

- *Stress echocardiography*

Fluoroscopy

Chest fluoroscopy, unlike the simple chest x-ray, uses a continuous beam to image movements of the thoracic region. This continuous x-ray beam is used for the identification of a paralyzed hemidiaphragm. For example, a hemidiaphragm that is paralyzed will move paradoxically and cranially, while a normal and unimpaired hemidiaphragm will be seen as moving caudally, or toward the spinal column.

Computed Tomography (CT)

Another imaging study is computerized Tomography (CT) Scans: CT scans take cross sectional images of the entire body. These images provide more information than x-rays. Computerized tomography is one of the most highly used diagnostic imaging procedures.

CT scans can be done with or without a contrast media. The CT scan facilitates the evaluation of abnormalities of the patient's lungs, mediastinum, pleura and chest wall, and the diagnosis of pulmonary emboli.

Similar to a simple chest x-ray, computed tomography images thoracic abnormalities and structures but with a more clear and refined image within multiple 10 mm thick cross sectional images. It is relatively inexpensive and highly available in the healthcare environment, however, its disadvantages include motion artifacts and compromised detail and clarity with some tissue.

High-resolution computed tomography, also referred to as HRCT, gives us a 1 mm thick cross sectional image typically during the patient's full inspiration in order to facilitate the best possible images of the airways, the lung's vasculature, the lung parenchyma; it is highly useful for detecting and evaluating obliterative bronchiectasis and interstitial lung disorders such as sarcoidosis, alveolitis and lymphangitic carcinomatosis, masses, infiltrates, and fibrosis. HRCT images can also distinguish between dependent atelectasis and other atelectasis.

Spiral or helical computed tomography, done while the patient holds their breath for about 10 seconds, gives us multiple images of the entire chest while the patient is moved gradually and continuously through the CT scanning device. Some of the advantages of spiral or helical computed tomography, when compared to the traditional and conventional CT, include less exposure to radiation, speed, its ability to produce three dimensional images and to create a virtual bronchoscopy with the help of specialized software. The most recent multi-detector CT machines allow for even more rapid scanning and imaging of thinner slices at higher resolution.

CT Angiography

CT angiography uses an intravenous radiopaque dye and it is particularly useful for the examination of the pulmonary arteries, the coronary arteries, the chambers of the heart, the flow of blood to the brain via the carotid arteries, and to perform concurrent balloon angioplasty, an embolectomy or an artherectomy. Its benefits, when contrasted with conventional angiography, include the fact that it is less invasive and more rapid than conventional angiography, and it provides high levels of accuracy.

An angiography allows for the evaluation of arterial abnormalities, such as arterial aneurysm, pulmonary embolism, or tumors, by injecting contrast medium in the patient.

A ventilation perfusion scan is an angiography to examine lung perfusion and an image of the distribution of ventilation through inhaling radiolabeled gas (xenon 133), which is useful in diagnosing pulmonary emboli.

MRI

An MRI study is a highly detailed evaluation of the chest, which includes the heart, major vessels, mediastinum, lungs, and chest wall. It is more expensive than other diagnostic imaging procedures. Contraindications to MRI include morbidly obese patients and patients with a device, such as cardiac pacemaker or intracranial aneurysm clips, dependent upon metallurgical composition.

Although this imaging is relatively limited in terms of pulmonary imaging, it is preferred for the detection of tumors, pulmonary hypertension and cysts, and also among patients with an intolerance to contrast dye when a pulmonary embolus is suspected.

The disadvantages of MRI include the time needed for this imaging test, the presence of cardiac and respiratory movements, and its contraindications for some patients. Among the advantages of MRI are the absence of bone artifacts, the lack of exposure to radiation, and its ability to provide superior images of the vascular structures.

Nuclear Scanning

Nuclear scanning techniques used to image the chest include:

- *Ventilation/Perfusion (V/Q) scanning*

- *A perfusion (Q) scan and*

- *Positron emission tomography (PET.)*

Ventilation/perfusion, or V/Q, scanning entails the injection of an intravenous radionuclide to assess perfusion and the inhalation of a radionuclide to assess ventilation. Specifically, areas of perfusion without ventilation and areas of ventilation without perfusion can be visualized with six to eight lung views.

This test is indicated when poor perfusion is suspected as can be the case with bronchial obstructions secondary to the aspiration of a foreign body, another bronchial obstruction, and an alveolar disorder such as consolidation, atelectasis, and emphysema.

A perfusion (Q) scan is done after the intravenous administration of radioactive technetium. This radioactive scan is indicated when an under perfusion of the pulmonary circulation is suspected. Such under perfusion can occur as the result of a tumor, a pulmonary embolism and/or pulmonary hypertension.

Normal ventilation and perfusion has a 1:1 ratio of blood and air in the alveoli; a pulmonary embolism leads to a V/Q ratio of >2: 1 which indicates that the ventilation is normal and the perfusion is absent or reduced; airway obstructions, such as that which can occur as the result of a atelectasis, have a V/Q ratio of 1 or <1: 2 or >2 because the perfusion is normal and the ventilation is absent or reduced.

Positron emission tomography or PET uses fluorodeoxyglucose to assess and measure the metabolic activity in tissues. It is used to determine the metabolism of the heart and the brain, to determine pulmonary perfusion and ventilation, to determine the size and extent of a myocardial infarction, and to metabolically stage tumors without the need for more invasive staging methods that involve, for example, a needle biopsy and a mediastinoscopy.

Position emission tomography (PET) creates images of metabolic tissues by injecting small amounts of a radioactive tracer into the patient. The PET detects metabolic cellular changes and can help to identify rapidly growing cells like those associated with lung cancer.

Ultrasonography

Ultrasonography is often used to facilitate procedures such as thoracentesis and central venous catheter insertion but it is also used for the diagnosis of a pulmonary disorders such as a pleural effusion.

OTHER DIAGNOSTIC TESTS

Other commonly used diagnostic tests are:

- *Transillumination*
- *Oxygen challenge test*
- *Pulmonary function tests*

Transillumination of the Chest

Transillumination is the shining of a light source through a bodily area or organ to assess for any abnormalities. Some of the areas that can be assessed using transillumination include the circulatory vessels, the chest, scrotum, and head of a neonate or preterm infant as well as the breasts of adult female patients.

Some of the respiratory system disorders that can be detected with transillumination, among young and premature infants, include the hydrocele, hydrocephalus, chest abnormalities such as a pneumothorax, and the collection of air around the heart. Transillumination to the head, for example, will have scattered light up when the Chun gun projects light and hydrocephalus is present.

Other abnormal findings can suggest:

- *Hydrocele:* This appears light red in color.

- *Pneumothorax:* The light reflects off the anterior chest wall when it penetrates the thin anterior wall.

- *Lesions and internal bleeding:* The area will be dark in color and even black in color.

The Oxygen Challenge Test

The transcutaneous oxygen challenge test (OCT) provides data relating to the degree of transcutaneous partial pressure of oxygen (PtcO2) in response to 1.0 FiO2. The transcutaneous partial pressure of oxygen (PtcO2) index can detect low flow secondary to circulatory failure and possibly a low cardiac output.

Pulmonary Function Tests

The results of a patient's pulmonary function tests are, in most cases, located in the respiratory therapy section of their medical record.

Pulmonary function tests involve having the patient perform a variety of both inspiratory and expiratory maneuvers using a number of specialized equipment. The test is performed in order to measure a patient's airflow, volumes/capacities, and gas diffusion. Often times these results will discover information that is relevant to whether or not the patient has an obstructive disorder, such as asthma or chronic obstructive pulmonary disease (COPD), a restrictive disorder which can include a variety of neuromuscular diseases, or a disorder or condition that affects the patient's gas diffusion.

These pulmonary function tests include:

- *Pulse oximetry*
- *Spirometry*
- *Compliance and airway resistance*
- *Lung volumes*
- *Broncho-provocation studies*
- *Exercise testing*

The most common forms of cardiopulmonary exercise testing are:

- *Exercise induced broncho-constriction testing*
- *Full cardiopulmonary exer-cise testing*
- *The Six Minute walk test*

Exercise testing is often used to diagnose exercise induced bronchoconstriction. This test entails the measurements of the FEV1 and FVC before beginning and after 5, 15, and 30 minutes of exercise on a cycle ergometer or treadmill when the heart rate is 80% of its predicted maximum rate. Exercise-induced bronchospasm is suspected when the FEV1 or FVC drops by ≥ 15% after exercise.

Computerized complete cardiopulmonary exercise testing (CPE) provides patient data in reference to oxygen consumption, carbon dioxide production, air flow, cardiac rate, and, often, arterial blood gas results while the patient is at rest as well as exercising while on a treadmill or using a bicycle ergometer.

This testing data differentiates between reduced exercise capacity and normal maximal exercise capacity. It also identifies the offending organ system associated with a patient's exercise intolerance and/or exertional dyspnea.

The Six Minute walk test is a nonspecific test of the patient's ability to ambulate at their own pace and rate for six minutes. This is a global function test, rather than a specific test for exercise intolerance and exercise capacity.

ASSESSING AND MONITORING AIRWAYS

ESTABLISHING AN AIRWAY

Depending on the patient's condition, there are a number of different airways that can be used when indicated during resuscitation. These airways include:

- *Bag valve masks*
- *Oral and nasopharyngeal airways*
- *Laryngeal mask airways (LMA)*

- *Esophageal-Tracheal tubes (Combitube)*
- *Endotracheal tubes*
- *Tracheostomy tubes*

Bag Valve Masks

Bag-valve-mask (BVM) devices can deliver 60 to 100% of oxygen when properly placed and properly used. The airway patency is ensured with the proper patient head position.

Oral and Nasopharyngeal Airways

Oral and nasopharyngeal airways are indicated when the patient is not conscious and experiencing a seizure, when the unconscious patient can potentially obstruct their airway with their tongue, and when a patient with an endotracheal tube is biting this tube. These airways are not indicated when the patient is conscious because it may lead to gagging, vomiting, and life-threatening aspiration. The two most common types of oropharyngeal airways are hollow centered and I beam types.

Oropharyngeal airways come in different sizes for both pediatric and adult patients. Proper sizing can be simply done by placing the airway against the patient's face and the end of the airway reaches the angle of the jaw. Airways that are too small push the tongue into the oropharynx rather than pulling the tongue forward as it should. An airway that is too large can lead to the blockage of the oropharynx. A properly sized and placed oropharyngeal airway should lift and move the tongue forward and enable suctioning.

Laryngeal Mask Airways (LMA)

These airways have an inflatable mask which forms a seal around the larynx that is connected to a modified endotracheal tube. This tube provides an alternative to the placement of an endotracheal tube or a Combitube, and they are relatively simple to insert, but they are not as secure as an endotracheal tube. Another advantage of these airways is the fact that they are more effective than bags to mask ventilation during resuscitation. They can be connected to mechanical ventilators, resuscitation bags, and anesthesia machines.

As with all artificial airways, respiratory therapists recommend the insertion of a specific type of airway, and they also recommend changes in airways so it is important for them to understand each airway, its indications, contraindications, advantages, and disadvantages.

Some of the indications for a laryngeal mask include use after CPR, when patients have a difficult airway that cannot be managed with an endotracheal tube such as when the patient is affected with asthma or an irritable airway because these airways lead to less coughing and bronchospasm than an endotracheal tube, when a patient's neck cannot be hyperextended for endotracheal tube placement, and when passage of an endotracheal tube needs a channel that can be provided with a laryngeal mask airway.

These tubes are contraindicated among patients who have gastro-esophageal reflux disease, when the patient has food contents in their stomach, as well as when the patient is conscious and resisting its placement. These tubes do not prevent aspiration and they can cause leakage of tidal volume gases from the mouth and into the stomach when mechanical ventilation pressures are greater than 20 cm of water.

Laryngeal mask airways are manufactured in various sizes. For example, a size 1 is used for neonates and infants weighing up to 11 pounds, size 4 is used for adults up to 154 pounds, and larger sizes are used for adults over this weight.

The steps for insertion of a laryngeal mask airway are:

1. *Deflate the lubricated mask and place it in the mouth.*

2. *Slide the mask into the oral pharynx behind the tongue.*

3. *Advance the mask until resistance at the opening of the larynx is felt.*

4. *Attach a syringe and inflate the mask so it seals the larynx.*

Placement is ascertained by hearing bilateral breath sounds when the lungs are inflated with a resuscitation bag.

Esophageal-Tracheal Tubes (Combitube)

A Combitube, which is a two lumen tube, can be placed in the trachea or the esophagus which is also referred to as an esophageal obturator airway. These tubes are used when endotracheal intubation is not successful and when the patient is unconscious and apneic. They are not used when endotracheal intubation is possible, when the patient has an intact gag reflex and is conscious, when the patient has esophageal pathology or trauma such as having swallowed a corrosive substance, or when this device is needed for more than 2 hours.

Some of the advantages of a Combitube include its relatively rapid and simple placement, its ability to prevent gastric contents from moving into the pharynx, and it can be inserted without any hyperextension of the neck or head.

Despite its advantages, some of its disadvantages are the risk of an upper airway tear during insertion, air leakage, and an unintended tracheal intubation.

The steps for insertion and placement are:

1. *Place the head in a neutral position, and then pull the jaw forward.*

2. *Insert it into the center of the mouth and slide forward until the black rings on the tube are at the patient's teeth.*

3. *Inflate both of the cuffs.*

The correct placement and position are determined by listening to breath sounds as a resuscitation bag, attached to the shorter endotracheal tube, is inflated.

Endotracheal Tubes

Endotracheal tubes offer superior and secure airways, particularly when a medical emergency occurs. It prevents aspiration, it permits direct suctioning, and it can be attached to mechanical ventilation. An endotracheal tube consists of an inflation tube, a pilot balloon, a one-way valve, a body, cuff, bevel, and a 15 mm outer diameter adapter at the proximal end.

These tubes come in different sizes to accommodate for all the age groups along the life span from size 4 mm to 14 mm outer diameter and 2.5 to 10 cm in terms of inner diameter; they can remain in place for a couple of weeks when needed. For example, an adult will use an 8.0 to 8.5 inner tube diameter. Pediatric tubes can have a constant diameter or a wide proximal end that tapers and narrows at the distal end. The selected tube should have a low pressure cuff and a large residual volume, unless contraindicated.

Endotracheal tubes are contraindicated when a patient is adversely affected with a neck injury that prohibits hyperextension of the head and neck, and/or oral surgery is being done.

Endotracheal tubes can be classified as:

- *Standard*

- *Wire reinforced, or armored, which prevent tube damage when bitten by the patient*

- *Performed tubes which are bent forward to keep the tube and anesthesia away from the patient's face and bent backward to keep the tube and anesthesia away from the patient's neck*

- *Guidable trigger tubes that have a ring that, when pulled, shortens the radius of the tube's curve*

- *Double lumen tubes which allow independent ventilation and they are useful during special procedures such as a pneumonectomy or a bronchoscopy*

- *High frequency jet ventilation tubes which accommodate for both standard and jet ventilators*

- *Oropharyngeal suctioning tubes which have built in suctioning catheters*

Some of the complications of endotracheal intubation include perforation of the pharynx or esophagus, bronchospasm, vocal cord injury, injuries from excessive cuff pressure, reflex bradycardia, hypotension, and a healthcare- or hospital-related infection as a result of this invasive procedure.

Endotracheal tubes are placed with a laryngoscope, either straight or curved of appropriate size, and the procedure is as follows:

- *Hyper-oxygenate the patient.*

- *Remove all foreign material including dentures from the patient's mouth.*

- *Guide the straight laryngoscope blade so it just passes the epiglottis but not too far because it can enter the trachea or esophagus, or guide the curved blade into the valecula.*

- *Lift the epiglottis and visualize the vocal cords, arytenoids, and esophagus.*

- *Place the tube into the right side of the patient's mouth and slide it into the trachea.*

- *Take the laryngoscope blade out.*

- *Inflate the cuff.*

- *Hyperventilate the lungs.*

The correct positioning and placement of endotracheal tubes is determined by palpating the tube as it moves through the larynx and into the trachea, auscultating bilateral breath sounds, determining the presence of condensation in the tube upon expiration, using capnography to check for the presence of carbon dioxide during exhalation, assessing a chest radiograph for proper placement, determining whether or not the 24 cm mark is at the adult's front central incisors, and determining if there is any asymmetrical chest movements, tracheal deviation, and/or crepitus. An esophageal detection device checks for the proper placement of the tube into the airway. Properly placed endotracheal tubes should be in the middle third portion of the trachea.

Tracheostomy Tubes and Devices

Like an endotracheal tube, a tracheostomy tube provides a secure airway, mechanisms for direct suctioning, a route for mechanic ventilation and the prevention of the aspiration, and it can also be used among patients affected with facial trauma and upper airway obstructions. It can be used for long term treatment. These tubes are placed with surgery.

Tracheostomy tubes include a standard tracheostomy tube and fenestrated tubes. A fenestrated tracheostomy tube should replace a standard tracheostomy tube when the patient is able to spontaneously breathe when not ventilated. The inner cannula is removed and the cuff is deflated to enable the patient to spontaneously breathe; the inner cannula is replaced and the cuff is inflated when the patient returns to mechanical ventilation.

The sizes of tracheostomy tubes are the same as those of endotracheal tubes. They range from 4 mm to 14 mm in terms of their outer diameter and from 2.5 to 10 cm in terms of their inner diameter.

Obstructions of the lumen can occur as the result of the cuff sliding over the tip of the tube, secretions, and tube placement in subcutaneous tissues. The placement of a tracheostomy tube is assessed and determined by auscultating for equal and bilateral lung sounds, chest radiography, and measuring exhaled carbon dioxide. No breath sounds should be heard over the stomach area.

The correct cuff pressure should be no more than 25 mm Hg or 35 cm of water. The following actions are taken when the patient experiences a complete or partial airway obstruction with a tracheostomy tube:

- *Rule out a plug obstruction by deflating the cuff and suctioning the patient; if a suctioning catheter cannot be passed, remove the inner cannula and clear the mucus plug.*

- *Withdraw the tube and allow the patient to breathe through the stoma if these interventions are unsuccessful because it is possible that the tube has entered soft tissue.*

Difficult Airway Recognition

Maintaining a patent airway, the primary and most basic of human needs, is facilitated by the respiratory therapist by addressing a number of different considerations and interventions such as:

- *Proper patient positioning*

- *Emergency resuscitation and ventilation*

- *Suctioning*

- *Placing and maintaining an artificial airway*

- *Noninvasive and noninvasive mechanical ventilation*

Some neonates, infants, and children have medical and anatomical abnormalities that make the establishment of an airway quite challenging. Some examples of these abnormalities include airway infections, laryngeal obstructions, craniofacial trauma, and craniofacial malformation. Some alternatives for the management of the airway for these challenges are:

- *Anterior commissure intubation*
- *Flexible fiber optic intubation*
- *Emergency tracheotomy*

Anterior Commissure Intubation

Anterior commissure intubation is indicated among patients with a craniofacial abnormality such as Treacher Collins syndrome, Pierre Robin syndrome, or hemifacial microsomia. Anterior commissure intubation is done with a special laryngoscope called a Holinger anterior commissure laryngoscope, which is a tubular, rigid laryngoscope that facilitates the visualization of the endolarynx so the endotracheal tube can be passed in the scope with long alligator forceps.

Flexible Fiber Optic Intubation

Flexible fiber optic intubation is done with a flexible fiber optic bronchoscope which has advantages over the use of a standard laryngoscope to the endolarynx and it also facilitates nasotracheal intubation when a patient is affected with a disorder such as muscular dystrophy (MD), a craniofacial abnormality, or a mass in the airway.

Emergency Tracheotomy

Emergency tracheotomy should be done after an airway is secured, however, this is not always possible because of severe craniofacial malformations, an obstructed larynx, or severe trauma. In these cases, mask ventilation, a cricothyroidotomy, or a tracheotomy with local anesthesia may be indicated.

Other lesser used intubation techniques that can be used when the airway is difficult include retrograde tracheal intubation, finger intubation of the trachea, using a Neustein or Bullard laryngoscope, and intubation using a laryngeal mask airway.

STANDARD INTUBATION

In addition to the kinds of intubation procedures discussed immediately above, there are two other types of intubation can be performed for neonates, infants, and children:

- *Nasotracheal intubation*
- *Endotracheal intubation*

Nasotracheal Intubation

When the child no longer needs endotracheal intubation and is stable, nasotracheal intubation can be indicated.

The patient is prepared with medications to decrease inflammation and swelling. Some of these include oxymetalozine to decongest the airway and a vasoconstrictive spray like phenylephrine. The size of the endotracheal tube is often the same or about one size smaller than that which was used for their endotracheal intubation.

After the tube is lubricated, it is passed into the nose until one half of the tube is in place. An assistant will then hold the already placed endotracheal tube toward the left side of the mouth until the glottis is exposed. When the nasal tube is in the hypopharynx, the tube is held with a McGill forceps or an otologic alligator forceps and then advanced while the older tube is being gradually removed.

The depth of the tube is determined with the following formula:

The depth of the endotracheal tube in cm = 15 + Age in Years + 3

Some of the contraindications associated with nasotracheal intubation are facial/oral trauma, abnormal clotting, thrombocytopenia, hemorrhage, a basilar skull fracture, and choanal atresia.

Endotracheal Intubation

Endotracheal tubes are inserted and placed into the trachea through the mouth; however, at times it can be placed through the nose. These tubes have low and high volume balloon cuffs. In the past, cuffed tubes were only used for children over eight years of age and adults; however, they are now used among young children and infants.

Endotracheal tubes secure an adequate airway, prevent aspiration, permit suctioning of the lower respiratory tract, and facilitate mechanical ventilation among patients in need of prolonged durations of mechanical ventilation.

Placement requires proper positioning, as discussed above, and the use of laryngoscope, either straight or curved, of appropriate size. The procedure is as follows:

- *Hyper-oxygenate the patient*

- *Remove all foreign material including dentures from the patient's mouth*

- *Guide the straight laryngoscope blade so it just passes the epiglottis but not too far because it can enter the trachea or esophagus, or guide the curved blade into the valecula*

- *Lift the epiglottis and visualize the vocal cords, arytenoids, and esophagus*

- *Place the tube into the right side of the patient's mouth and slide it into the trachea*

- *Take the laryngoscope blade out*

- *Inflate the cuff*

- *Hyperventilate the lungs*

The correct positioning and placement of endotracheal tubes is determined by palpating the tube as it moves through the larynx and into the trachea, auscultating bilateral breath sounds, determining the presence of condensation in the tube upon expiration, using capnography to check for the presence of carbon dioxide during exhalation, assessing a chest radiograph for proper placement, and determining if there are any asymmetrical chest movements, tracheal deviation, and/or crepitus. An esophageal detection device checks for the proper placement of the tube into the airway. Properly placed endotracheal tubes should be in the middle third portion of the trachea.

Some of the complications of endotracheal intubation include perforation of the pharynx or esophagus, bronchospasm, vocal cord injury, injuries from excessive cuff pressure, reflex bradycardia, hypotension, and a healthcare- or hospital-related infection as a result of this invasive procedure.

Equipment Selection

The equipment that is used for intubation can be easily remembered with the MSMAID pneumonic as listed below:

M: Monitors including ECG, ETco2 detectors, pulse oximetry, blood pressure monitors, and a stethoscope

S: Suctioning equipment like a suctioning machine, catheters without a relief valve, sterile catheters for the endotracheal tube, and a Yankauer catheter

M: Machines such as the ventilator and the bag and mask

A: Airways and airway supplies such as artificial airways, laryngoscopes, infant or pediatric alligator forceps, Kolodny or McGill forceps, and 1 inch tape for securing the airway

I: Intravenous access

D: Drugs for anesthesia and drugs for resuscitation

Post-Intubation Tube Placement Verification

After intubation, the cuff is inflated using a 10 mL syringe and less than 30 cm H2O; often, properly sized tubes need less than 10 mL of air to create the correct pressure.

Tube placement is then checked and verified using a number of different methods including:

- *Inspection of the chest for its symmetrical rise*

- *Auscultation of the lungs for good breath sounds bilaterally without any gurgles in the upper abdomen*

- *Using an esophageal detector device*

- *A chest x-ray*

- *CO_2 detection with capnography or a CO_2 detection device*

ADVANCED INTUBATION

Some of the special advanced intubation techniques include:

- *Cricoid pressure*

- *Using tube changers*

- *Using specialty laryngoscopic visualization devices*

- *Intubation through a Laryngeal Mask Airway (LMA)*

Cricoid Pressure

Cricoid pressure of the neck, also referred to as the Sellick maneuver, is sometimes used to prevent regurgitation and to better visualize the glottis during endotracheal intubation.

Until 2010, the American Heart Association recommended the use of cricoid pressure during resuscitation and during emergent oral endotracheal intubation, however, now it is not recommended during routine intubation except during a cardiac arrest.

Some of the complications of cricoid pressure are displacement of the esophagus laterally, glottic compression, esophageal rupture, increases in peak pressures, and reductions in tidal volume.

Tube Changers

Tube introducers, or tube changers, are often referred to as gum elastic bougies. These semi-rigid stylets are useful when the epiglottis can be visualized but the laryngeal opening is not.

Tube introducers are moved along the under surface of the epiglottis and, then, more easily into the laryngeal opening. When in place, an endotracheal tube is then advanced over the tube introducer. The tube is rotated at 90 degrees in a counter clockwise manner if it is caught in the right aryepiglotic fold.

Specialty Laryngoscopic Visualization Devices

Specialty laryngoscopic visualization devices and special intubation techniques are highly useful after laryngoscopy has not been successful and when conditions such as those detailed above lead to a difficult airway. Some special laryngoscopes are:

- *Mirror and video laryngoscopes*

- *Fiber optic scopes and optical stylets*

Video and mirror laryngoscopes facilitate looking around the tongue to provide better visualization of the larynx.

Flexible fiber optic scopes and optical stylets are highly useful when a patient has abnormal anatomy. Fiber optic scopes are more difficult to use, when compared to a video or mirror laryngoscope, and they also tend to be more problematic when dealing with secretions and blood.

LMA

Intubation can be done by passing an endotracheal tube through an LMA. This technique, like the others above, takes practice and the mask must be properly placed and positioned over the laryngeal inlet in order to be effective.

Cuff Management

Simply stated, tracheal tube and laryngeal mask cuff pressure should be maintained at the lowest possible level that is necessary for ensuring air sealing. Some of the complications associated with high cuff pressures include:

- *Endothelium damage*
- *Inflammation*
- *Nerve damage*
- *Ulceration*
- *Ischemia*
- *Necrosis*

Pressures that are too low cause leaks and the potential for the aspiration of oropharyngeal or supraglottic secretions.

Many guidelines and evidence based procedures recommend that the "ideal pressure" is the minimal occlusion volume that is needed to seal the airway. Some others recommend that the pressure be maintained lower than the venous perfusion pressure and between 16 and 24 cm of H_2O. Nonetheless, monitoring of the cuff pressure should be done in a continuous and ongoing manner according to the specific healthcare facility's policy and procedure.

AIRWAY CLEARANCE TECHNIQUES

The removal of respiratory secretions can be done with a number of different procedures and techniques including:

- *Postural drainage*
- *Using mechanical devices for airway clearance*
- *Percussion*
- *Secretion removal with suctioning*
- *Vibration*

Postural Drainage, Percussion, and Vibration

Bronchopulmonary secretions can be removed by performing postural drainage, percussion, and vibration. These three techniques are often referred to as pulmonary physiotherapy or pulmonary hygiene.

Postural drainage is done using the force of gravity to remove secretions when the patient is positioned in a manner that drains all the lobes of the lung. For example, the patient is placed in the following positions to drain the upper lobe of the lung, the lower lobe of the lung and lingular areas.

The Upper Lobe

- *Anterior bronchus: Supine with a pillow under the knees*

- *Apical bronchus: Semi-Fowler's position and then leaning to the right, to the left, and then forward*

- *Posterior bronchus: Up at a 45 degree angle and up against a pillow at 45 degrees on the left side and then on the right side*

The Middle Lobe

- *Medial and lateral bronchus: A 30 degree Trendelenburg position and turned slightly to the left or a 14 to 16 inch elevation of the foot of the bed and turned slightly to the left*

The Lingula

- *Apical bronchus: Prone position and a pillow under the patient's hip*

- *Medial bronchus: A 45 degree Trendelenburg position and turned on the right side or an 18 to 20 inch elevation of the foot of the bed and turned on the right side*

- *Lateral bronchus: A 45 degree Trendelenburg position and turned on the left side or an 18 to 20 inch elevation of the foot of the bed and turned on the left side*

- *Posterior bronchus: A 45 degree prone Trendelenburg position and a pillow under the patient's hip*

- *Superior and inferior bronchus: A 30 degree Trendelenburg position and turned slightly to the right or a 14 to 16 inch elevation of the foot of the bed and turned slightly to the right*

Percussion is performed by placing a cup over the area and doing percussion to remove secretions. Each area is percussed for at least one minute while the patient is holding his or her breath. Vibration is performed by laying the hand on the area and applying rapid vibrating movements while the patient is deeply exhaling. Percussion and vibrations are applied to areas after the patient is positioned for postural drainage, as follows.

The Upper Lobe

- *Anterior bronchus: Just under the clavicles over the anterior chest*

- *Apical bronchus: Over the shoulder blades to the clavicle*

- *Posterior bronchus: Over the shoulder blades on both sides*

The Middle Lobe

- *Medial and lateral bronchus: From the axillary fold to the mid-anterior chest and over the lateral right chest and the anterior right chest*

The Lingula

- *Apical bronchus: The lower third of the posterior rib cage bilaterally*

- *Medial bronchus: The lower third of the left posterior rib cage*

- *Lateral bronchus: The lower third of the right posterior rib cage*

- *Posterior bronchus: The lower third of the posterior rib cage bilaterally*

- *Superior and inferior bronchus: The left axillary fold to the mid-anterior chest*

Airway Clearance Using Mechanical Devices

Positive expiratory pressure (PEP) therapy is done with the use of a mask or a mouthpiece and a one-way valve that is connected to a manometer, set at between 10 and 20 cm H2O. It provides the patient with expiratory pressure during the middle of the expiration phase thus moving secretions from peripheral airways to the larger airways for removal.

For this form of chest physiotherapy, the patient is sitting and instructed to hold his or her breath for approximately three seconds after a slow inspiration. Then, as the patient slowly exhales through the mouthpiece and resister, the forced exhalation mobilizes respiratory tract secretions. This is done from 10 to 20 times per session.

There are also devices that combine vibrations, as previously discussed, with positive expiratory pressure (PEP) therapy.

Secretion Removal with Suctioning

Suctioning devices include suction catheters and a vacuum source. Suction catheters are made of rubber or plastic and they are made in different sizes. The largest possible diameter suction tube should be used to prevent clogging. The sizes reflect the outer diameter of the catheter in the measurement known as French (Fr.) They range in outer diameter from 5 Fr to 16 Fr. The outer diameter should never be more than ½ of the inner diameter of the artificial airway tube. The recommended sizes, according to age and body build, are below:

- *Neonate: 5, 6 and 8 Fr*

- *Pediatric patients from 18 months to 8 years of age: 8 to 10 Fr*

- *Adults over 16 years of age: 10 to 16 Fr*

The outer diameter of a catheter can be calculated by:

Outer diameter = Catheter Fr size x 0.33

The inner diameter of the catheter can be calculated by:

Inner diameter in mm = $\dfrac{\text{Fr size - 2}}{4}$

The three major types of suctioning catheters are a bevel cut catheter with two side holes, a ring tipped catheter with several holes around it, and a curved tipped, or Coude, catheter which is curved to facilitate advancement into either the right or left bronchus.

Open airway suctioning is defined as suctioning when the patient is able to breathe room air and closed airway suctioning is defined as suctioning that is done with the oxygen supply connected. The latter is the preferred method of suctioning, particularly when the patient is at risk for hypoxia relating to the suctioning.

Endotracheal and tracheostomy suctioning entail surgical asepsis and sterile technique; other forms of suctioning are clean procedures using medical asepsis techniques. The most commonly occurring complication associated with suctioning is hypoxia. This hypoxia can be prevented by keeping the suctioning episodes as brief as possible and by oxygenating the patient. Suctioning is discontinued when hypoxia occurs.

Vacuum devices are most typically wall mounted central vacuum systems which have regulators with off, full suction, and alternative settings that can be adjusted according to the patient's needs. Portable vacuum systems are used when central vacuum systems are not available.

This equipment is set up using the following steps.

1. *Connect the regulator to the suction regulator outlet*

2. *Connect a collection bottle that can contain at least 500 mL onto the regulator*

3. *Connect one end of the vacuum tube to the collection bottle and the other end to the suction catheter when suctioning is to be done*

4. *Adjust the negative pressure to the desired level*

When the suctioning equipment is not working correctly, the respiratory therapist should perform troubleshooting and, when this is not successful, this equipment should be immediately removed from service and sent to the biomedical equipment department, or another department as indicated in the healthcare facility's policies and procedures.

Some troubleshooting tips are determining if:

- *The vacuum system is correctly plugged into an outlet*

- *The vacuum system is turned on and set to the desired negative pressure*

- *The connected collection bottle is tightly connected without any leaks*

- *The tubing and the vacuum tubing are tightly connected*

- *There is any kinking, coiling, or obstruction in the tubing or suctioning catheter*

- *The collection bottle is filled to its capacity*

ADMINISTERING AND MONITORING SPECIALTY GASES

SPECIALTY GASES

GAS CYLINDERS

Although it is highly recommended that all gas cylinders are labeled, only E cylinders have mandatory color coding to differentiate among the various medical gases. The following colors are used for the following gases.

- *Green:* Oxygen

- *White:* The international color for oxygen

- *Yellow:* Air

- *Brown:* Helium

- *Brown and Green:* Helium and oxygen

- *Light Blue:* Nitrous oxide

- *Red:* Ethylene

- *Orange:* Cyclopropane

- *Gray:* Carbon dioxide

- *Gray and Green:* Carbon dioxide and oxygen

Because there is no way to see into a cylinder, respiratory therapists must be able to calculate how long a cylinder will last as based on the ordered gas flow and the flow factor (L/psig) for the particular cylinder size. The L/psig for each type of cylinder size is, as below.

- *E Cylinders: 0.28 L/psig*

- *H Cylinders: 3.14 L/psig*

- *K Cylinders: 3.14 L/psig*

- *D Cylinders: 0.16 L/psig*

- *M Cylinders: 1.36 L/psig*

- *G Cylinders: 2.41 L/psig*

Using the cylinder L/psig and the flow rate, the amount of time that the gas will last is calculated using the below formula. The minutes of expected flow are equal to:

$$\frac{\text{The gauge pressure in psig x The cylinder L/psig}}{\text{The liter flow}}$$

REGULATORS

Regulators combine a flow meter and a reducing valve, both of which are discussed immediately below.

Reducing Valves

Reducing valves lower and reduce the pressure in manifold, gas cylinder, and bulk oxygen storage systems. The two basic types of reducing valves are singe stage and multiple stage reducing valves.

Connectors

High pressure hose connectors connect flow meters, oxygen appliances, and high pressure hoses. They too have safety features which permit only the proper connections.

Flow Meters

Flow meters regulate the flow of gas. These flow meters have safety features that allow them to only be connected to the correct regulator, the correct high pressure hose, and the correct reeducating valve.

Flow meters can be backpressure compensated and non-backpressure compensated. The three basic types of flow meters are:

- *Pressure uncompensated flow meters*
- *Backpressure compensated flow meters*
- *Bourdon flow meters*

Backpressure compensated flow meters can be identified with the following steps.

1. *Turn the flow meter off.*

2. *Plug the flow meter into the working gas outlet.*

3. *Observe the float or ball. It is backpressure compensated when the ball or float bounces.*

The standard of care indicates that backpressure compensated flow meters should be used for all patients and all situations with the exception of transport situations when a non-compensated backpressure flow meter is used.

AIR / OXYGEN BLENDERS

Air/oxygen blenders, also referred to as air/oxygen proportioners, are used when high pressure gas of 50 psig is indicated and when the percentage of oxygen to air has to be adjusted. They are capable of changing this oxygen to air blend, or combination, from 21% to 100%.

OXYGEN CONCENTRATORS

Oxygen concentrators are used primarily by patients who are in the home. These concentrators deliver low flow oxygen. The two basic types of oxygen concentrators are a molecular sieve oxygen concentrator and a semipermeable plastic membrane oxygen concentrator.

Molecular sieve oxygen concentrators deliver oxygen to the patient through a flow meter after room air is moved by a compressor through sodium aluminum silicate in the form of zeolite pellets that remove nitrogen and water vapor. The percentage of oxygen delivered has an inverse relationship with the delivered flow. For example, the percentage of oxygen is about 92% to 95% when the flow in liters per minute is from

1 to 2 L/min and the percentage of oxygen is about < 85% when the flow in liters per minute is > 6 L/min.

Semipermeable plastic membrane oxygen concentrators deliver oxygen to the patient after room air is passed through a vacuum pump that removes excesses of water vapor with a condenser. External humidification systems are not needed when a semipermeable plastic membrane oxygen concentrator is used.

Unlike the molecular sieve oxygen concentrator, semipermeable plastic membrane oxygen concentrators deliver only 40% oxygen.

AIR COMPRESSORS

Compressors are necessary whenever high pressure gases, other than oxygen, are needed. The three types of compressors are rotary type compressors, diaphragm type compressors, and piston type compressors. All three filter room air, filter out excessive water vapor, and are operated with electricity.

TYPES OF SPECIALTY GASES

Some of the specialty medical gases are:

- *Nitric oxide*

- *Helium oxygen mixtures*

- *Hypoxic and hypercarbic gas mixtures*

- *Isoflurane*

Nitric Oxide

Nitric oxide (NO) diffuses through the alveolar membrane to the smooth where it increases the levels of cyclic guanosine monophosphate which, in turn, relaxes them. Nitric oxide therapy is used for respiratory disorders such as:

- *Persistent pulmonary hypertension of the neonate*

- *Adult respiratory distress syndrome*

- *Chronic obstructive pulmonary disease*

Nitric oxide for neonates with persistent pulmonary hypertension reduces pulmonary artery pressure, vasodilates the blood vessels, it reduces the shunt fraction, and it increases PaO2.

Caution must be exercised when using nitric oxide. When nitric oxide comes in contact with oxygen it forms NO2 which can lead to a serious acute lung injury like pulmonary edema and pneumonitis. Also rebound hypertension can occur when the patient is weaned off nitric oxide therapy so continuous monitoring is indicated.

Helium Oxide

Helium, the second lightest of all elements, has a low density of 0.179 g/L which makes it less dense than air, nitrogen, and oxygen, and it has a high viscosity of 188.7 UP which makes it more viscous than nitrogen and air but just slightly lower than that of oxygen.

According to the principles of Poiseuille's and Graham's laws, a gas of lower density will have a higher flow than gases with a higher density with pressure remaining constant and, therefore, less pressure is needed to maintain flow with an obstruction.

Helium oxygen mixtures, also referred to as heliox, are used to treat upper and lower airway obstruction and they decrease the work of breathing. This specialty gas, although not the treatment for airway obstruction disorders, does decrease the work of breathing until the treatment of the underlying cause can be rendered.

Helium oxygen mixtures come in different concentrations. For example, it may come in an 80% helium and 20% oxygen concentration or a 70% helium and 30% oxygen concentration.

Hypoxic and Hypercarbic Gas Mixtures

Hypoxic gases have less than 21% oxygen; hypercarbic gases and hypoxic gas combinations are used for respiratory disorders based on the principles that carbon dioxide is powerful vasoconstrictor and that oxygen is a powerful vasodilator. Based on these principles, respiratory therapists are able to alter the systemic blood flow and the pulmonary blood flow with the manipulation of the pulmonary vascular resistance using this specialty gas.

Hypoxic and hypercarbic gas mixtures are used for the treatment of neonates and infants with congenital heart disorders such as hypoplastic left sided heart syndrome and single ventricle syndrome.

Hypoxic gases are delivered with a mechanical ventilator or an oxygen hood. The oxygen is set to deliver 21% oxygen and then nitrogen and humidification are added. Hyberbaric gases are also delivered with a mechanical ventilator or an oxygen hood and carbon dioxide and humidification are added.

Close monitoring is essential in order to prevent suffocation. A highly sensitive oxygen analyzer is used and it must be capable of detecting very low oxygen concentration of about 17% to 18%. The low oxygen alarm must remain set and never turned off.

Isoflurane

Isoflurane, similar to other low dose halogenated specialty agents like halothan, desflurane, enflurane, and sevoflurane, can be used alone or in combination with nitrous oxide as an inhaled anesthetic agent during labor and delivery.

Although this anesthetic agent has been found to increase maternal oxygen levels and uterine blood flow, it can also cause complications. It can lead to significant maternal and fetal CNS depression as well as maternal Mendelson syndrome, a form of pneumonitis that occurs as the result of a combination of a general anesthetic agent and undigested food in the stomach. The signs and symptoms of Mendelson syndrome include cyanosis, tachycardia, fever, chest pain, and respiratory distress.

MANAGING VENTILATION AND OXYGENATION

OXYGEN SUPPLEMENTATION

Oxygen supplementation is indicated when there is documented or suspected hypoxemia. This evidence is collected with blood gas results, pulse oximetry results, and the clinical signs and symptoms associated with hypoxemia.

When the Spo2 is less than 95% and/or the Pao2 is less than 80 mm Hg, hypoxemia is present. For the neonate, a Pao2 and a Spo2 less than 90% indicate the need for resuscitation and the initiation of oxygen therapy.

The clinical manifestations of hypoxia among infants and young children are tachypnea and tachycardia. Later signs include bradycardia, apnea and decreased respiratory rate, nasal faring, retractions, irritability, restlessness, grunting, and a "frog leg" which indicates fatigue and muscle flaccidity. Cyanosis is considered a late sign among infants.

The settings begin and are adjusted through the therapy according to the Pao2 and the Spo2. Some of the recommended flow rates for different oxygen administration devices are listed below.

- *Nasopharyngeal Catheter: Flow rate between 0.25 and mL/minute with 100% to maintain the FIO2 at about 0.24 and 0.35 as indicated by the patient's inspiratory flow rate. These catheters are not very often used today.*

- *Nasal Cannula: Typically less than 3 L/min flow rate.*

- *Oxygen Masks: A flow rate of between 6 and 10L/min to provide an FIO2 of 0.35 to 0.5.*

- *Partial Rebreathing Reservoir Mask: 6 to 15L/min is usually enough to maintain the FIO2 up to 0.6.*

- *High Flow Nasal Cannula: A maximum of 2 L/min.*

- *Oxygen Tent: Low to moderate oxygen concentrations of less than 45% can be achieved with an oxygen tent and flow rates of more than 10 L/ min yields an oxygen concentration of less than 50% even with the source oxygen at 100%.*

- *Oxygen Hood: The flow rate should be greater than 7 L/min and, in most cases, and a flow rate of 10 to 15 L/min is sufficient for infants and children.*

- *Incubators: Incubators have one oxygen connection for low to moderate oxygen concentrations of about 40% and another for higher oxygen concentrations of about 100%. Oxygen analyzers increase the oxygen flow and decrease the oxygen flow according to these analyses.*

The ordered amount of oxygen should be based on the current arterial blood gases or the pulse oximetry reading. The amount of supplemental oxygen should maintain the Pao2 between 60 and 80 mm Hg and 92% to 100% saturation without any signs of oxygen intoxication, or toxicity.

The lowest possible Fio2 that maintains an acceptable Pao2 should be given; a Fio2 > 60% is not used except under dire life-threatening emergencies. A Fio2 < 40% can be delivered with a nasal cannula or simple face mask; a Fio2 > 40% requires use of an oxygen mask with an inflated reservoir. Humidification is used with oxygen therapy to moisten secretions and to facilitate easier production.

The Components of Mechanical Ventilators

The components of a mechanical ventilator include:

- *Input power*

- *Power conversion and transmission*

- *Controls including the control circuit, control variables and waveforms,* *phase variables, modes of ventilation, conditional variables. and spontaneous versus mandatory breaths*

- *Output*

- *Alarm systems including input power alarms, control* *circuit alarm. and output alarms*

Input Power

Ventilators are classified as electrically powered and pneumatically powered. At the current time, however, most ventilators have both pneumatic and electrical power. The electrically driven aspect of the ventilator delivers gas and the pneumatic aspect of the ventilator provides the driving forces of the ventilator.

Power Conversion and Transmission

Power conversion and transmission, referred to as the drive mechanism, includes the compressor and the output control valves. Internal and external compressors generate gas flow and the output control valves control the flow of gas from the compressor.

The several types of compressors are the pneumatic diaphragm, the electromagnetic poppet valve, or solenoid, the pneumatic popper valve, and the electromagnetic proportional valve which controls flow by modifying the size of the valve opening when there is a need to pattern inspiratory flow.

Controls

The Control Circuit

The control circuit is the "brain" of the ventilator that makes decisions to regulate the output control and the drive mechanism. Ventilator control circuits can be a mechanical control circuit, a fluidic control circuit, or an electrical control circuit. These circuits can be further classified as open or closed loop circuits; both loops have an input of flow setting, pressure, and volume and an output of the desired outcome in terms of oxygenation.

Control Variables and Waveforms

Control variables include flow, pressure, and volume. These variables, collectively, create motion; the waveforms include the pressure, volume, flow, and time waveforms. Dual control of the inspiratory phase can be accomplished when the ventilator being used can switch from one control variable to another, as based on a specific condition during the inspiratory phase.

Phase Variables

Phase variables are used during mechanical ventilation to initiate, maintain, and end of the ventilatory phase. The phases of the respiratory cycle are:

I.   *The transition, or change, from expiration to inspiration*

III.   *The transition from inspiration to expiration*

II.   *Inspiration*

IV.   *Expiration*

Trigger phase variables initiate inspiration during Phase I; the limit variable is a preset value that limits the pressure, volume, and flow before the end of expiration. Infants are typically pressure limited. Cycle variables end the inspiratory phase; time, flow, volume, and pressure can all be used as cycle variables.

Modes of Ventilation

Modes of ventilation can be simply described as a pattern of phase variables and control for both spontaneous and mandatory breaths.

Conditional Variables

Conditional variables occur when the ventilator initiates and selects a particular pattern of control and phase variables for each breath. For example, an alternative pattern is selected and initiated when a conditional variable does not reach its preset value and the same pattern is used when the conditional variable reaches its preset value.

Spontaneous vs. Mandatory Ventilation

Simply defined, a mandatory breath is one that is imitated or terminated by the ventilator and a spontaneous breath is defined as one that the patient initiates and terminates. Spontaneous breaths can be assisted with pressure support or unassisted all together.

Output

Output and output waveforms result from the changes and the magnitude of the changes in flow, pressure, and volume over the course of the inspiration.

Alarm Systems

The purpose of alarms and alarm systems is to alert the respiratory therapist of changes in the patient status and/or changes in the functioning of the mechanical ventilator. Alarms are set to monitor all the variables that are involved in the mechanics of breathing, namely: volume, pressure, flow, and time

Input alarms are activated when an electrical ventilator loses electrical power; pneumatic ventilators have input alarms that alert us to a significant reduction or complete loss of oxygen pressure or compressed air. Control circuit alarms signal problems such as a breakdown of the microprocessor as well as some lack of incompatibility of control settings such as would occur when the settings establish an inverse I:E ratio.

Lastly, output alarms signal the provider when there is some variable that is outside of its normal range. These ranges can be established by the respiratory therapist, automatically set as based on control settings and still more may be set as a default by the manufacturer.

Of the many alarms, the most common are the:

- *High and low baseline pressure*

- *High and low exhaled tidal volume*

- *High and low mean airway pressure*

- *High and low exhaled minute volume*

- *High and low respiratory rate*

- *Too long or too short duration in terms of inspiratory time*

- *Too long or too short duration in terms of expiratory time*

- *High and low FIO2 alarm*

- *High and low gas temperatures*

- *Exhaled oxygen tension*

- *Exhaled carbon dioxide tension*

TYPES OF VENTILATORS

There are several types of ventilators:

- *Pneumatic respirator*

- *Electrical respirator*

- *Fluidic ventilator*

- *Microprocessor volume cycled respirator*

Pneumatic ventilators operate with electricity which is provided by a wall outlet or a battery. These ventilators are particularly helpful when a ventilator-dependent patient is transported and when there is an external disaster in the community because it can operate with a battery. Electrical ventilators do not have this advantage.

Electrical ventilators are primarily volume cycled ventilators and as such a preset volume of air is delivered to the patient regardless of their condition and respiratory functioning.

Fluidic ventilators, used among the neonates and pediatric patients, are powered pneumatically and they have fluidic controls. These controls are highly sensitive to obstructions and changes in other ventilator settings.

Microprocessor ventilators are controlled with computer microprocessors and driven with electricity. These ventilators deliver all modes of ventilation and they also have other features including spirometry measurement, which is highly useful when the patient is being weaned from the ventilator. They also automatically calculate airway resistance, dynamic and static lung compliance, and they have a continuous display of critical assessment data like volume, flow, pressure, and PEEP. In addition to these benefits, microprocessor ventilators also have automated problem identification which is visually displayed on the unit.

All ventilators differ in term of their setup, maintenance, troubleshooting, and settings, so it is highly important that all respiratory therapists are highly knowledgeable about the particular ventilator that they are using.

CONTINUOUS MECHANICAL VENTILATION

Mechanical ventilation can be delivered with a tracheostomy tube, an endotracheal tube, and with noninvasive methods such a face mask and nasal cannula for CPAP and BiPAP. Briefly stated, continuous mechanical ventilation delivers air under pressure that keeps the alveoli open during inspiration and prevents alveolar collapse during expiration. It improves oxygenation and gas exchange, it decreases the work of breathing, and it forces and increases the expansion of the lungs.

The common modes of ventilation are:

- *Positive end expiratory pressure (PEEP): Preset pressure during spontaneous inspiration*

- *Continuous positive airway pressure (CPAP): Preset positive pressure during spontaneous inspiration*

- *Bilevel positive airway pressure (BiPAP): Preset positive pressure during spontaneous inspiration and spontaneous expiration*

- *Assist control: Preset tidal volume and rate*

- *Synchronized intermittent mandatory ventilation: Preset tidal volume and rate*

- *Independent lung ventilation: Double lumen endotracheal tube that is used among patients with one sided lung disorders*

- *High frequency ventilation: Small amounts of gas at rate from 60 to 3,00 cycles/min and used among children*

- *Volume assured pressure support ventilation: Preset minimal tidal volume per breath*

- *Inverse ratio ventilation: Lengthens inspiratory phase and used for hypoxemia refractory to PEEP*

- *Pressure support ventilation: Preset pressure during spontaneous inspiration*

Microprocessor volume cycled ventilators have graphic displays that combine any two of the following for comparison:

- *Time*
- *Volume*
- *Flow*
- *Pressure*

For example, plateau and peak pressure are best displayed with comparing time and pressure; air trapping is best seen by comparing time to flow; lung inflection is determined by comparing volume and pressure.

Patients who are on microprocessor mechanical ventilation can also have their work of breathing assessed which further adds to the respiratory therapist's assessment and observation of the patient's shortness of breath, the use of accessory muscles, and signs of fatigue. The work of breathing can be decreased when the ventilator is set to minimize the inspiratory flow and the negative pressure; ideally, the inspiratory flow and sensitivity should be adjusted after a pressure/volume loop is performed.

Airway resistance measurements are important in order to determine how well or difficult it is for the patient to move tidal volume through the airways and they are also helpful for determining whether or not aerosolized bronchodilating medications are effective.

Airway resistance among normal adult patients without any pulmonary disorder should be 0.6 to 2.4 cm water/L/sec with spontaneous breathing; normal infants who weigh 3 kg, for example, are expected to have 30 cm water/L/sec. Airway resistance is increased when patients are using an endotracheal tube; the resistance is also increased in an inverse relationship to the size of the tube. For example, the smaller the tube, the greater the airway resistance.

The airway resistance is mathematically calculated using these formulas.

Peak flow in liters/sec =
$$\frac{\text{Peak flow in L/min}}{60 \text{ seconds}}$$

Airway resistance =
$$\frac{\text{Peak airway pressure – Plateau pressure}}{\text{Peak flow in liters/sec}}$$

INTERMITTENT POSITIVE PRESSURE BREATHING (IPPB)

Intermittent positive pressure breathing consists of the delivery of a gas to a spontaneous breathing patient under positive pressure with either an aerosol or humidity for intermittent periods of time no more than 20 minutes in duration.

IPPB creates a greater than normal vital capacity because of this positive pressure; this positive pressure also contacts the airways, the chest, and the lungs.

The advantages and effects of intermittent positive pressure include:

- *Increased tidal volume*

- *Increased mean airway pressure*

- *Beneficial changes in the inspiratory/expiratory (I:E) ratio*

- *A decrease in the work of breathing*

IPPB is indicated for a number of disorders and conditions such as to increase sputum clearance, to collect a sputum sample, to facilitate the patient's coughing, to deliver aerosol medications, to treat atelectasis when other methods have not been successful, and to manage patients with pulmonary edema.

Intermittent positive pressure is contraindicated among patients affected with a tracheoesophageal fistula, active and untreated tuberculosis, singulation, nausea, air swallowing, a bleb as seen with a chest x-ray, intracranial pressure of more than 15 mm Hg, and hemodynamic instability.

The steps for initiating intermittent positive pressure are listed below:

1. *Connect the electrical unit into the socket or the pneumatic unit to the compressed air or oxygen outlet*

2. *Set the sensitivity to – 1 cm*

3. *Adjust and set the flow*

4. *Set the peak pressure between 10 and 15 cm H2O*

There are passive intermittent positive pressure treatments and active intermittent positive pressure treatment. Patients receiving a passive treatment are advised to relax and let the air fill the lungs until the pressure is achieved. The patient is then instructed to hold their breath before passive exhalation. The goals of passive intermittent positive pressure treatments are to decrease the work of breathing and to allow medications to enter the lungs and the airways.

Active intermittent positive pressure treatments, on the other hand, involve the patient breathing with the IPPB machine; this form of treatment is often used to prevent atelectasis. Patients often need coaching and practice to adjust their breathing patterns until they are synchronous with the IPPB. Therapists can also adjust flow, sensitivity, volume, pressure, the fractional concentration of inspired oxygen, and the auto PEEP (positive end expiratory pressure) to facilitate this synchrony. Respiratory therapists modify these treatments as based on their responses to the therapy.

Some of the complications associated with intermittent positive pressure include a hospital-acquired infection, hyperoxia when 100% oxygen is delivered, hypocarbia, hemoptysis, air trapping, over-distended alveoli, hyperventilation, decreased venous return, pneumothorax, impacted secretions when adequate humidity is not delivered, and increased airway resistance.

ALTERNATIVE MODES OF VENTILATION

Some alternative modes and methods of ventilation that can be used as based on the patient's condition and the desired outcome(s) include:

- *Volume targeted ventilation*
- *Neurally adjusted ventilation*
- *Pressure ventilation*
- *Ventilatory control ventilation*
- *Airway pressure release ventilation*
- *Ventilatory assist/ control ventilation*
- *High frequency ventilation*

Volume Targeted Ventilation

Volume targeted ventilation, also referred to as volume control ventilation, consists of a constant flow rate and a constant tidal volume. As a result of these constants, the peak inspiratory pressures will vary when there are changes in resistance and compliance.

Pressure Ventilation

Pressure ventilation can be classified as positive pressure ventilation or negative pressure ventilation. Positive pressure ventilation employs high external pressures to drive gases into the lungs with lung inflation. Negative pressure ventilation, on the other hand, creates a vacuum in the airway that expands the thorax and creates decreases in pleural pressure lower than the airway, thus allowing gases to enter the lungs.

This form of ventilation does NOT require the use of an artificial airway, therefore, it is often referred to as a noninvasive type of ventilation.

Airway Pressure Release Ventilation

Airway pressure release ventilation is a form of continuous positive airway pressure ventilation. This form of ventilation provides continuous positive airway pressure ventilation in addition to pressure release settings.

This alternative form of ventilation is used among patients who have intrapulmonary shunting as the result of acute respiratory distress syndrome or respiratory distress syndrome and who have not responded successfully to other treatments.

High Frequency Ventilation

High frequency ventilation is indicated when a smaller tidal volume and/or a higher respiratory rate is needed and cannot be delivered with regular volume cycled ventilators. Although it is primarily used among neonates and infants, it is sometimes used for adults who are undergoing a procedure such as a laryngoscopy or bronchoscopy.

High frequency ventilation can be delivered in three different ways as listed below.

- *Using a high frequency oscillation ventilator*

- *Using a conventional ventilator set to a maximum rate of 150/min*

- *Using a high frequency jet ventilator*

Neurally-Adjusted Ventilation

Neurally-adjusted ventilation is defined as a type of ventilation that permits the patient full neurological control over the over the ventilator's magnitude, triggering, and timing supports regardless of any changes in the patient's respiratory mechanics, neurological and chemical respiratory drive, and/or muscular function.

This form of ventilation is used in combination with a special nasogastric tube that has electronic sensors to obtain data about the diaphragms activity as well as the timing and pressure of delivered ventilations.

This form of ventilation is used among patients who are adversely affected with the work of breathing, gas trapping, and auto PEEP. It is not affected or altered leaks or secretions so, hypocapnia and auto-cycling can be eliminated among neonates and young infants.

Ventilation Control

In the control mode, it is the respiratory therapist and the ventilator that have complete control over the patient's respiratory functioning.

All ventilations are given at a preset and established pressure, volume, frequency, and rate. This type of ventilation requires that the patient is sedated and paralyzed to prevent any asynchrony between the patient's respiratory efforts and the ventilator's preset deliveries.

This form of ventilation may be necessary when the patient needs extreme control. A complication of asynchrony with this form of ventilation is pneumothorax which most often occurs among patients affected with asthma or acute respiratory distress syndrome.

Ventilator Assist/Control Mode

The ventilator assist/control mode allows the ventilator and the respiratory therapist to maintain most control over the patient's respiratory functioning; however, it also gives the patient the ability to voluntarily use their own respiratory drive to trigger the ventilator to deliver breaths of a preset pressure or volume.

The ventilator is preset with inspiratory flow rate, frequency, and volume or pressure, and it maintains support with each breath with this form of ventilation. When the patient is able to breathe at the established rate, the ventilator does not initiate it, however, when the patient does not initiate the breath within the established period, the ventilator delivers the breath at the pre-set rate.

Noninvasive Modes of Ventilation

Non-invasive ventilation, also referred to as noninvasive positive pressure ventilation, is defined as ventilation without the use of an endotracheal or tracheostomy tube. These patients are ventilated with a nasal or full face mask that delivers CPAP and BiPAP.

Non-invasive ventilation is used among patients who need short term support and capable of spontaneous respiration. Unstable patients are not candidates for this ventilation. For example, patients affected with sleep apnea, COPD, asthma, heart failure, and pulmonary edema, when stable, may be a good candidate for short term non-invasive ventilation.

Continuous Positive Airway Pressure (CPAP)

Continuous positive airway pressure (CPAP), a noninvasive ventilation method, delivers environmental air which is above the atmospheric pressure during the patient's spontaneous breathing. For this reason, patients with CPAP must be able to adequately and sufficiently inhale oxygen and exhale carbon dioxide. The patient's blood pressure, cardiac rate, respiratory rate, tidal volume, and minute volume should be stable.

CPAP is contraindicated among apneic patients who, instead, require mechanical ventilation. CPAP is similar to PEEP in terms of its effects and purpose but it has its advantages over PEEP because CPAP does not lead to the same venous return reduction.

CPAP pressures are increased and decreased in small increments of 2 to 5 cm of water when CPAP is initiated. The patient is monitored for any signs and symptoms of fatigue including decreased maximum inspiratory pressure, decreased vital capacity, decreased tidal volume, an increased PaCO2, and increased respiratory and/or cardiac rate.

CPAP delivery devices include a mask and nasal prongs. Face masks can be full or partial; a full face mask is indicated for patients who are mouth breathers. A partial nasal mask covers only the nose and it enables the wearer to more freely eat, drink and talk. It also provides the wearer with the ability to breathe through the mouth should the CPAP machine malfunction and to release excessive pressure through the mouth.

CPAP masks are fitted for the patient. A poor seal with gas leakage and insufficient pressure occur when a mask is too large; masks that are too small can lead to facial mars and the delivery of uneven pressure over the face. Nasal prongs can be used with patients who breathe through their nose. They are preferred by many patients particularly those who cannot tolerate a mask over their face.

Bilevel (BiPAP) Ventilation

Bilevel ventilation consists of two levels of positive pressure. The baseline pressure is greater than zero and the peak pressure is established as based on the goal for the tidal volume. Each of these two levels can be adjusted according to patient's subjective reports, the result of the arterial blood gases, the breath sounds, and the vital signs. Up to 15 L/min of oxygen can be added to the port, the humidifier or the BiPAP machine, as indicated. This amount of oxygen is determined by the patient's SpO2.

Bilevel BiPAP machines can be for expiratory positive airway pressure, inspiratory positive airway pressure, spontaneous ventilation, and spontaneous timed ventilation.

The steps for initiating bilevel ventilation, in correct sequential order, are:

1. *Setting the expiratory positive pressure*

2. *Adjusting the expiratory positive pressure to achieve the desired tidal volume*

3. *Setting the inspiratory positive airway pressure*

4. *Adjusting the inspiratory positive airway pressure*

ADJUNCT TECHNIQUES

Some of the adjunct techniques that are used in respiratory care among the pediatric population are:

- *Lung recruitment maneuvers*
- *Patient positioning*
- *Extracorporeal gas exchange*
- *Extracorporeal membrane oxygenation (ECMO)*
- *Carbon dioxide removal*

Lung Recruitment Maneuvers

Lung alveolar recruitment is used for acute respiratory distress syndrome. PEEP improves the volume of lung aeration and oxygenation. It also allows the use of a lower Fio2.

Most maintain that the least amount of PEEP to maintain adequate arterial oxygen saturation is indicated when the patient is adversely affected with acute respiratory distress syndrome. A PEEP between 8 and 15 cm H2O is typically adequate, however, at times it may have to be increased to more than 20 cm H2O in severe cases.

Patient Positioning

Recent research has indicated that a prone position facilitates lung recruitment and improved oxygenation among patients with respiratory distress syndrome.

Extracorporeal Life Support Circuits

Extracorporeal life support circuits consist of a cannula, a heat exchanger, post membrane pressure monitor, O2 blender, membrane oxygenator, pre-membrane pressure monitor, a pump, fluid chamber, a heparin source, and a venous reservoir.

Extracorporeal life support, simply stated, is an artificial lung. This supportive treatment exchanges gas(es) across the membrane depending on the surface area, the thickness of the membrane, the type of gas, and the partial pressure difference on each side of the membrane, which is referred to as the driving pressure.

The driving pressure varies according to the type of gas. For example, the driving pressure of oxygen 720 mm Hg because the sweep gas is 100% oxygen, the pO2 outside of the membrane is about 760 mm Hg and the venous pO2 is 40 mm Hg. It is calculated as follows:

760 mm Hg – 40 mm Hg = 720 mm Hg

The driving pressure of oxygen is 720 mm Hg; the driving force of carbon dioxide is 45 mm Hg. Despite the low driving force of carbon dioxide, the silicone in the membrane is six times more permeable in terms of carbon dioxide than it is with oxygen.

Two extracorporeal gas exchange techniques are:

- *Extracorporeal membrane oxygenation (ECMO)*

- *Carbon dioxide removal*

Extracorporeal Membrane Oxygenation (ECMO)

Extracorporeal membrane oxygenation (ECMO) is used for the treatment and support of acute respiratory distress syndrome, neonatal pneumonia, severe sepsis, persistent pulmonary hypertension of newborns, and for congenital diaphragmatic hernias. It is indicated when infants are not able to be adequately ventilated and/or oxygenated with a mechanical ventilator.

The procedure for this technique entails heparinization followed with the circulation of the infant's blood through a large diameter catheter from the internal jugular vein into a membrane oxygenator to remove any carbon dioxide and the to add oxygen. This oxygenated blood is then recycled back into the internal jugular vein (venovenous ECMO) or the carotid artery (venoarterial ECMO.) The former is referred to as venovenous ECMO and the latter is referred to as venoarterial ECMO. Venoarterial ECMO is indicated when ventilatory support, in addition to circulatory support, is needed as is the case with severe sepsis.

The flow rates are adjusted and maintained to achieve the desired O2 saturation and blood pressure.

The complications associated with ECMO include hematologic problems like hemolysis, neutropenia and thrombocytopenia, thromboembolism, cholestic jaundice, air embolus, and neurological disorders such as seizure and stroke.

ECMO is contraindicated among neonates and infants less than 34 weeks of gestation and less than 2 kg in weight because of the risks associated with the systemic heparinization that is need to do this procedure.

Carbon Dioxide Removal

As stated previously, the silicone in the membrane for extracorporeal treatments is six times more permeable in terms of carbon dioxide than it is with oxygen. The carbon dioxide is transferred across this membrane as a result of this permeability rather than on the blood flow rate or the thickness of the blood film thickness. Instead, the removal of carbon dioxide occurs as a function of the driving pressure, the surface area of the membrane, and the gas flow rate.

MONITORING

Respiratory therapists monitor and assess patients in a continuous and ongoing manner in order to determine:

- *The severity of the lung disease*
- *Airway pressures and volumes*
- *Gas exchanges*
- *Ventilator graphics*
- *Ventilator waveforms*
- *Ventilator-patient interaction*
- *Effects of mechanical ventilation on cardiac function*

- *Pulmonary mechanics*
- *Pulmonary compliance*
- *Airway resistance*
- *Vital capacity tests*
- *The I:E ratio*
- *Tidal volume*
- *Minute volume*

Severity of Lung Disease

The severity of the lung disease is determined with a wide variety of methods including the history, physical examination, invasive tests, noninvasive tests, and data collected with other studies such as laboratory tests and imaging studies.

Primary modifications of testing for the neonate, infant, and young child are based on the fact that these populations are unable to cooperate with the respiratory therapist's requests. Many young patients will also need chloral hydrate with a dosage of 50 to 75 mg/kg for sedation. Although this sedating medication is relatively safe, it can lead to respiratory distress when the oxygen saturations are compromised. Other modifications include the use of the face mask for testing. The mask resistance and the mask's dead space must be as low as possible to get accurate testing results.

Creative approaches that reassure pediatric patients and elicit their cooperation, when at all possible, should include a child-friendly environment, the use of play to test, the presence of the parents, and simple explanations appropriate to the patient's age and level of development.

Airway Pressures and Volumes

The primary pulmonary function tests are gas volume as flow rates into and out of the lungs. The rate of gas flow for the pediatric population is measured with pneumotachometer which is also referred to as a pneumotach. Of the several types of pneumotachometers, the Fleish pneumotach is the most commonly used. These devices can have a variable or fixed orifice and they all operate on the same principle which is that an obstruction of gas will lead to a drop in pressure.

A second type of pneumotach is the heat transfer pneumotachometers are also known as hot wire anemometers and thermistor type devices. These units consist of a heated thermistor that is cooled as air passes around it. When the gas moves past the wire and cools, it cools in proportion to the amount of gas and this lends itself to a flow reading which is then converted into volume. These devices, when attached to a microprocessor, measure, calculate and display various patient values.

Gas Exchanges

Changes of pressure in the airways pushes gas into and out of the lung for both spontaneous breathers and those who are mechanically ventilated. Mechanically ventilated patients receive gases because the ventilator applies positive pressure and they rid the body of gases with a recoiling of the chest wall and lungs. Despite the fact that expiration is referred to as a passive maneuver, it is, in reality, an active process that requires energy. Spontaneous breathers inhale when sub atmospheric pressure is created in the thorax and chest as the muscles of ventilation and the falling diaphragm expand the chest volume.

Trans-pulmonary pressure is the difference between airway pressure and plural pressure. This pressure moves gases.

Ventilator Graphics

A variety of ventilator graphics can be selected based on the clinical judgment of the respiratory therapist and the needs of the patient. For example they can select any two of the following:

- *Time*
- *Flow*
- *Pressure*
- *Volume*

For example, plateau and peak pressure are best displayed with comparing time and pressure; air trapping is best seen by comparing time to flow; lung inflection is determined by comparing volume and pressure.

Ventilator Waveforms

Waveform graphics include waveforms for flow, pressure, volume, and time. The analysis and interpretation of these waveforms allow the respiratory therapist to perform a number of different assessments and determinations such as:

- *Assessing the effects of administered bronchodilators*
- *Detecting equipment malfunctions*
- *Determining the appropriate PEEP level*
- *Assessing inspiratory termination criteria during pressure support ventilation*
- *Confirming mode functions*
- *Evaluating the adequacy of inspiratory time in pressure control ventilation*

- *Detecting the presence and rate of continuous leaks*

- *Detecting auto-PEEP*

- *Determining patient-ventilator synchrony*

- *Assessing and adjusting trigger levels*

- *Measuring the work of breathing*

- *Adjusting the tidal volume and minimizing over distension*

Pressure waveforms can be rectangular and exponential; flow waveforms can be rectangular, exponential, sinusoidal, or an ascending ramp and a descending ramp; volume waveforms can be sinusoidal or an ascending ramp.

Ventilator-Patient Interaction

Patient Synchrony

Some of the recommendations to improve patient synchrony include coaching relating to altering the breathing pattern among older children and by adjusting the flow and sensitivity controls on the unit.

Enhancing Oxygenation

A number of factors are assessed and considered in order to enhance the patient's oxygenation. For example, despite the fact that most patients are kept in the supine position, some patients may benefit more in terms of oxygenation when they are placed in the Fowler's or the semi-Fowler's position. When a supine and upright position does not effectively improve the level of oxygenation and promote more comfortable breathing, the patient can be turned to one side.

Respiratory therapists can also recommended changes in the oxygen administration level to prevent hypoxemia. The goal of oxygen therapy is to maintain the SpO2 greater than 90% and the PaO2 levels between 60 to 90 torr with some exceptions.

The formula to determine the desired FIO2 is as follows:

$$\frac{\text{Current FiO2 x Desired PaO2}}{\text{Current PaO2}}$$

Improving Alveolar Ventilation

Alveolar ventilation is a function of respiratory rate and tidal volume even when the minute volume remains stable. People without respiratory disorders typically have very little alveolar dead space, however, those with respiratory disorders have alveolar dead space that must be accommodated for in order to maintain alveolar ventilation.

Adjusting the I:E Settings

The inspiratory flow may have to be adjusted to modify the I:E ratio. Additionally, the expiratory time may have to be increased to allow for more complete exhalation when the patient has auto PEEP.

Modifying the Modes of Ventilation

Respiratory therapists often recommend changes in the modes of ventilation as based on the patient's current needs. For example, the respiratory therapist may recommend one of the following modes:

- *Control ventilation for apneic patients*

- *Assist/control ventilation to allow the patient to breathe on their own*

- *Intermittent mandatory ventilation to synchronize the patient and the breaths delivered by the ventilator*

- *Synchronous intermittent mandatory ventilation to enable the patient to trigger off tidal volume despite the fact that there is a preset interval*

- *Pressure support ventilation when the patient can deliver a ventilator breath*

- *Pressure control ventilation which delivers pressure-limited and time-cycled breaths*

- *Airway pressure release ventilation when an acute respiratory distress syndrome patients has not responded satisfactorily to constant volume ventilation*

Monitoring and Adjusting Alarm Settings

Under most circumstances the alarm are set from less than 10% to more than 10% of the patient's normal ventilator settings. Some ventilators can also alarm when the I:E ratio is 1:1 or less.

Adjusting Ventilator Settings Based on Ventilator Graphics

As previously stated, respiratory therapists can assess and make recommendations in term of ventilator graphics such as waveforms. For example, the respiratory therapist can determine the effects of administered bronchodilators and the appropriate PEEP for the patient and, as a result of these assessments, the respiratory therapist will make adjustments.

Changing the Type of Ventilator and Breathing Circuitry

There are several types of ventilators and there are several modes of ventilation, all of which were fully discussed above. As with all other aspects of respiratory care, respiratory therapists are responsible and accountable for changing and recommending changes in terms of type of ventilator and the mode of ventilation.

Reducing Auto-PEEP

Respiratory therapists must be able to assess and determine why the patient is air trapping when on mechanical ventilation. In essence, this occurs when expiratory time is too brief for the full and complete exhalation of the tidal volume. This brevity of expiratory time can be related to bronchospasm, excessive secretions, and a large tidal volume that cannot be expired. The recommendations for each of these are the administration of a bronchodilator, suctioning and the reduction of tidal volume along with an increase in the expiration time, respectively.

Pulmonary Mechanics

Pulmonary mechanics determinations are made with these and other tests:

- *Maximal inspiratory pressure testing*
- *Maximal voluntary ventilation testing*
- *Maximal expiratory pressure testing*
- *Vital capacity testing*

Maximal Inspiratory Pressure

Respiratory disorders can include diseases and disorders that interfere with the adequate functioning of the muscles that are essential to respiratory functioning and oxygenation.

Measures of maximal inspiratory pressure and measures of maximal expiratory pressure are particularly useful for this assessment and to aid in a differential diagnosis particularly when respiratory muscle impairment is suspected and when the results of the spirometry testing indicates the possibility of restriction as evidenced with a reduced vital capacity (VC), a low maximal voluntary ventilation, (MVV) lowered forced expiratory volume in one second (FEV1), lowered total lung capacity, and/or reduced forced vital capacity (FVC.)

Maximal inspiratory and maximal expiratory pressure tests measure the strength of the respiratory muscles during expiration and inhalation. Maximal inspiratory pressure tests measure the pressure that occurs when a maximal inspiration pushes against a closed system typically at residual volume. Maximal expiratory pressure tests measure the pressure that occurs with a maximal expiration.

These tests are also useful for monitoring the patient's current condition with a known disorder such as a neuromuscular disorder, heart failure, and chronic lung conditions.

Maximal inspiratory pressure (MIP) reflects the pressure that is expended by the patient when he or she exerts a maximal inspiration against a closed system mouth piece; it is the highest possible voluntary negative pressure that the patient can exert. The MIP is most useful for assessing the strength of the diaphragm and other muscles of inspiration.

Maximal inspiratory pressure is typically measured and documented as the residual volume (RV) because lung volume and inspiratory muscular strength have an inverse relationship. A normal MIP for males can, for example, be calculated and estimated with this arithmetic equation:

MIP = 142 - (1.03 x Age in Years) cm H_2O.

Maximum Expiratory Pressure

The maximum expiratory pressure, or MEP, reflects the strength of the abdominal breathing muscles and the other muscles of expiration. The MEP, also referred to as the maximum expiratory force, is measured by having the patient exhale with as much possible effort against a mouthpiece. The maximum patient value closely approximates the total lung capacity for the patient.

Maximum Voluntary Ventilation

The maximal voluntary ventilation (MVV) is the total amount of air that the patient can exhale while performing deep and rapid breathing for twelve seconds. A difference between the predicted and actual measured maximal voluntary ventilation can be caused by a less than adequate effort on the part of the patient, a lack of sufficient neuromuscular strength and reserve, and abnormal respiratory muscular mechanics.

The maximal voluntary ventilation test measures the total volume of exhaled air after twelve seconds of deep and rapid breathing; a predicted maximal voluntary ventilation is the forced expiratory volume (FEV1) multiplied by 40 or 35. When there is a discrepancy between the predicted maximal voluntary ventilation and the measured maximal voluntary ventilation it can indicate impaired respiratory mechanics in addition to a neuromuscular impairment.

Pulmonary Compliance

Pulmonary or lung compliance reflects the degree to which the lungs and thorax easily; it is impacted by lung elasticity and pulmonary volume. Low pulmonary compliance occurs when the recoil of the lungs is decreased and the lungs become stiff, as often occurs among the elderly and patients affected with edema, the absence of surfactant among neonates, asthma, pneumothorax, restrictive lung disorders, pulmonary fibrosis, and pneumonia.

Normal lung compliance can be decreased in patients with acute respiratory distress syndrome (ARDS) or with significant atelectasis. Diseases that cause the lung to become stiff, which include pulmonary fibrosis and acute respiratory distress syndrome, are associated with loss of lung compliance (CL), which is suggested with rising plateau pressures on patients who are mechanically ventilated.

Airway Resistance

Airway resistance is the measurement, in terms of cm H2O, of opposition to the flow of air, in terms of L/min, through the tracheobronchial tree and the bronchopulmonary system. Airway resistance impedes air flow with a number of conditions such as cigarette smoking, asthma, and COPD.

Vital Capacity Tests

Vital capacity tests also monitor a patient's neuromuscular strength, but, unlike other tests, vital capacity tests depend on the cooperation of the patient. A patient, in most cases, should have a vital capacity of at least 15 ml/kg of body weight.

The I:E Ratio

The I:E ratio is the ratio of the inspiration duration and the expiration duration of time. A normal I:E ratio is 1:2; and it is extended, for example, to 1:3 or more when airflow is obstructed and insufficient such as occurs with chronic obstructive pulmonary disease and asthma. Some sources cite the normal I:E ratio as 1:2 to 1:4. Abnormal I:E ratios are often accompanied with abnormal breathing patterns such as Biot's respirations, Cheyne-Stokes respirations, and Kussmaul's respirations.

Adult patients who are on mechanical ventilation with normal respiratory mechanics should have an I:E ratio of 1:3. Those with impaired respiratory mechanics, such as patients affected with asthma and chronic obstructive pulmonary disease should have an I:E ratio of at least 1:4 to limit the auto PEEP.

I:E ratios can be mathematically calculated using Ti and Te; Ti and Te can be calculated using the I:E ratio.

Tidal Volume

Tidal volume is the volume of air that is inhaled and exhaled during the patient's normal inhalation and their exhalation without the exertion of any extra effort. Normal adults have a tidal volume of about 500 mL during each inspiration or approximately 7 mL/kg of body weight.

Minute Volume

Minute volume is the volume of air that is exhaled from the lungs in one minute, which is referred to as the expired minute volume, or the volume of air that is inhaled into the lungs in one minute, which is referred to as the inhaled minute volume.

Other Volume Measurements

- *Expiratory reserve volume* which is the greatest amount of air that can be exhaled after the end expiratory phase

- *Forced expiratory volume* which is the forced vital capacity in context with the number of seconds that this measurement lasted

- *Inspiratory reserve volume* which is the greatest amount of air that can be inhaled from the end inspiratory position

- *Residual volume* which is the amount of gas left to reside in the lung at the end of a forceful, maximal exhalation

Effects of Mechanical Ventilation on Cardiac Function

Despite the benefits of mechanical ventilation in terms of gas exchange and decreased work of breathing, mechanical ventilation can affect cardiac functioning. Some of the effects of mechanical ventilation on cardiac function include:

- *Alterations in the systemic venous return to the right ventricle of the heart*

- *Reduced circulatory volume*

- *Decreased cardiac contractility*

VENTILATION STRATEGIES

Some of the special strategies that respiratory therapists employ with the pediatric population include:

- *Liberation from mechanical ventilation*

- *The prevention of ventilator induced lung injury*

- *Lung protective ventilation*

LIBERATION FROM MECHANICAL VENTILATION

Protocols

The American Association for Respiratory Care (AARC) supports the use of respiratory therapist implemented protocols, which follow a pre-established set of physician orders and interventions. With these protocols, the respiratory therapist can initiate, refine, and discontinue treatments based on these protocols and patient criteria or indicators. You can read them at the provided hyperlink.

Weaning

The five methods of weaning are:

1. *Ventilator discontinuance*

2. *Intermittent ventilator discontinuance*

3. *Regular SIMV weaning*

4. *Irregular SIMV weaning*

5. *Weaning with pressure support ventilation*

Respiratory therapists recommend the initiation of weaning and they also recommend one or the above methods of weaning as well as changes in the weaning method as based on the patient's continuous assessment and monitoring during the weaning process.

Ventilator Discontinuance

Patients who are awake, stable, and alert are good candidates for this type of weaning, particularly when they have been ventilated for only a relatively brief period of time. Ventilator discontinuance is abrupt; weaning occurs at the same time that the ventilator is discontinued. The patient is abruptly moved from the ventilator provision of all the minute volume to none at all. For obvious reasons, the patient must be monitored continuously until stable and then every 5 to 10 minutes thereafter. These assessments minimally include the vital signs and the patient's respiratory mechanics.

The procedure entails suctioning the patient, disconnecting the ventilator and then providing the patient with an oxygen and aerosol mix through a T piece connected to a reservoir. After 20 minutes, the arterial blood gases, end tidal carbon dioxide, pulse oximetry, and other tests as indicated are performed. Depending on the results of these tests, the patient can be either extubated or continue with this weaning process.

Intermittent Ventilator Discontinuance

Intermittent ventilator discontinuance may be the first choice of weaning or it can be initiated when a patient has not remained stable during abrupt ventilator discontinuance, as discussed immediately above.

This method is the same as ventilator discontinuance with the exception of the fact that this method has periods of weaning interspersed with periods of rest. As the patient continues to progress, the periods of weaning increase and the periods of rest decrease.

Regular Synchronous Intermittent Mandatory Ventilation (SIMV) Weaning

Synchronous intermittent mandatory ventilation (SIMV) is not only a method of weaning, it is also a ventilator mode. This weaning method is more gradual than ventilator discontinuance and it is used primarily for patients who have been ventilator dependent for a prolonged period of time in order for their respiratory muscles to strengthen after a period of time when they were not used because the patient had been on mechanical ventilation.

The patient remains on the ventilator with SIMV setting and the need for constant monitoring is lessened because the alarms remain activated. The procedure entails reducing the SIMV rate by 2 every minute on a set schedule of about 20 minutes. The patient is then assessed in terms of their blood gases, their spontaneous minute volume, and their respiratory mechanics. As this weaning process continues, the patient should get to the point where they can be extubated or place on a T piece.

(SIMV) Weaning

Irregular synchronous intermittent mandatory ventilation (SIMV) should be recommended and initiated when regular synchronous intermittent mandatory ventilation (SIMV) has not been successful.

The weaning method involves the reduction in the SIMV rate until the patient can no longer tolerate any further reductions. At this point, the SIMV is maintained at this level until the patient is able to tolerate further reductions. At times the SIMV should be increased to a higher level when the patient is experiencing poor tolerance.

One of the most commonly occurring reasons for a failure of this weaning method is resistance to breathing through the breathing circuit. This obstacle may be overcome with the use of a T piece, and when this is still not successful, the pressure support ventilation weaning method should be recommended and initiated.

Weaning with Pressure Support Ventilation

As just stated, the pressure support ventilation mode is used among patients who are not able to successfully wean with the irregular synchronous intermittent mandatory ventilation (SIMV.)

This method of weaning entails the gradual reduction of the pressure support level on the ventilator in increments of 2 to 5 cm of water. When the patient is able to tolerate these decreases they can be extubated.

Regardless of the weaning method used, signs that the patient is not tolerating the weaning process include:

- *A significant increase or decrease in the respiratory rate*

- *Anxiety and agitation*

- *Tachycardia*

- *Cardiac arrhythmias*

- *Cyanosis*

- *Hypertension or hypotension*

- *Hyperoxemia*

- *Hypercarbia accompanied with acidemia*

PREVENTING VENTILATOR-INDUCED LUNG INJURY

Despite the high usefulness of mechanical ventilation, there are also complications that can lead to physiological damage, including lung damage.

Some of these complications include over distention of the alveoli, cardiovascular complications, oxygen toxicity, hypoventilation, hyperventilation, infection, patient ventilator asynchrony, airway complications, other cardiopulmonary system complications, and other complications that are not related to cardiopulmonary functioning.

Alveolar Over Distention

Alveolar over distention is the most commonly occurring complication that can occur as the result of mechanical ventilation. The causes of this over distention and their causes include:

- *Atelectrauma: Repeated closing and opening of the alveoli with low lung volume*

- *Barotrauma: High ventilating pressures*

- *Volutrauma: Large tidal volumes*

This over distention leads to complications including pneumomediastinum, pneumoperitoneum, pneumothorax, subcutaneous emphysema, increased work of breathing, increased anatomical dead space, a decrease in static lung compliance, and leaking around the endotracheal tube.

Some of the treatments for over distention include decreasing the tidal volume, decreasing PEEP, the use of a chest tube and using permissive hypercapnia when a leak is detected. Less traditional interventions that can also be used when the aforementioned interventions are not successful include high frequency oscillatory ventilation, high frequency jet ventilation and extracorporeal membrane oxygenation.

High frequency chest wall oscillation and vibratory PEP are two examples of mechanical and passive devices that are used for airway clearance and chest physiotherapy. These devices are primarily employed for patients with chronic hyper-secretive disease and cystic fibrosis.

High frequency chest wall oscillation effectively increases the clearance of tracheal mucous using a vest like device that is worn by the patient. When this un-stretchable vest is connected to the air pulse generator, it deflates and inflates on the patient's chest about 5 to 20 times a second and, with this rapid action, it facilitates the patient's cough which enables the dislodgment of retained secretions.

High frequency ventilation is indicated when a smaller tidal volume and/or a higher respiratory rate is needed and cannot be delivered with regular volume cycled ventilators. Although it is primarily used among neonates and infants, it is sometimes used for adults who are undergoing a procedure such as a laryngoscopy or bronchoscopy.

High frequency ventilation can be delivered in three different ways as listed below.

1. *Using a high frequency oscillation ventilator*

2. *Using a conventional ventilator set to a maximum rate of 150/min*

3. *Using a high frequency jet ventilator*

Cardiovascular Complications

Ventilator cardiovascular complications include a decreased venous return, decreased cardiac output, increased pulmonary resistance, and a reduction of myocardial blood flow. These complications, often occurring as the result of increases of the intra-thoracic pressures, can be prevented among neonates and other members of the pediatric population by increasing the circulating volume.

The treatments for ventilator cardiovascular complications include the use of vasopressor medications and the administration of carbon dioxide or a nitrogen oxygen mixture with less than 21% oxygen to reduce any left to right shunting, to slow pulmonary blood flow, and to increase pulmonary vascular resistance.

Oxygen Toxicity

Oxygen toxicity can result from oxygen supplementation therapy when the level of oxygen concentration is too high, when the duration of the therapy is prolonged and when the severity of lung disease is so severe that higher levels of oxygen concentration are necessary to preserve life.

A loss of consciousness can occur when the $PaCO_2$ is increased and the patient is hypoventilating. Continuous monitoring of the blood gases for oxygen and carbon dioxide levels and maintaining the PaO_2 level between 50 and 60 torr can prevent this O_2 induced hypoventilation.

High FIO_2 levels from high concentrations of oxygen are also associated with retinopathy of prematurity among infants with a low birth weight and also chronic lung disease.

Denitrogenation Absorption Atelectasis

Denitrogenation absorption atelectasis can occur when more than 80% oxygen is administered; retinopathy of prematurity, formerly referred to as retrolental fibroplasia, is blindness that can occur among premature neonates when the PaO2 is not maintained between 50 and 60 torr during the first week of life and between 50 and 70 torr after the first week of life.

Pulmonary O2 toxicity can also occur among patients who are given more than 50% oxygen for more than 72 hours. CNS abnormalities such as seizures and muscular tremors can occur when a patient is receiving 100% in a hyperbaric chamber.

Hypoventilation

Hypoventilation can occur when there is either an inadvertent disconnection from the ventilator or an accidental extubation. To prevent these complications, respiratory therapists and other healthcare providers must be careful when transporting and repositioning patients to avoid these accidents. Additionally, low pressure and/or disconnect alarms must be set and monitored.

Other possible causes of ventilator associated hypoventilation are the loss of pulmonary compliance and increased resistance, both of which cannot be detected with a low volume monitor unless it is at the airway connection

Hypoventilation and under ventilation can be prevented with the continuous monitoring of the patient's resistance, compliance, flow volumes, and pressure volumes.

Hyperventilation

Hyperventilation can also occur from a number of different causes including ventilator auto-cycling because of a leak, a faulty sensitivity setting, the presence of secretions, and when the patient's lung compliance improves as the result of surfactant administration and/or repositioning into a prone or supine position.

Hyperventilation in combination with low carbon dioxide among low birth weight infants can lead to cerebral vasoconstriction and a cystic brain lesion referred to as periventricular leukomalacia.

The complication, like so many other complications, can often be prevented with close monitoring and the use of alarms. Specifically, the patient must be monitored in terms of tidal volume, minute volume, sensitivity levels, and carbon dioxide.

Hospital Acquired Infections

The most commonly occurring hospital-acquired infections, formerly known as nosocomial infections, associated with ventilator use are pneumonia and respiratory distress syndrome. Basic infection control measures including standard precautions, special precautions, maintaining asepsis and hand washing are essential to the prevention of hospital acquired infections, including those related to mechanical ventilation.

According to the National Guideline Clearing House, the following interventions are indicated for patients with mechanical ventilation in order to prevent ventilator associated pneumonia:

- *Elevation of the head of the bed*
- *Maintaining cuff pressure in the endotracheal tube between 20-25 mmHg*
- *Circuit changes*
- *Use of heated humidifiers and heat and moisture exchangers*
- *Providing oral care with chlorhexidine and water-soluble mouth moisturizer*

- Secretion removal with specially designed endotracheal tubes

- Kinetic bed therapy

- Sedation reduction

- Assessment of weaning readiness with brief weaning trials

Patient Ventilator Asynchrony

Patient ventilator asynchrony can lead to auto PEEP, respiratory alkalosis, increased work of breathing, and hyperventilation, as discussed above.

Airway Complications

Some of the airway complications associated with intubation and mechanical ventilation are:

- Glottic injuries like glottis stenosis, erosion and edema

- Tracheal injuries such as tracheomalacia, tracheal dilation, tracheoinnominate artery fistula, and tracheal erosion

- Airway obstructions as the result of plugs and kinking of the endotracheal and/or connection tubing

- Vocal cord injuries

Other Cardiopulmonary System Complications

These complications include:

- Pulmonary interstitial emphysema

- Pneumothorax

- Bronchopulmonary dysplasia

Other Complications

Other possible ventilator associated complications are increased intracranial pressure, periventricular leukomalacia, renal impairment, fluid retention, and inter-ventricular hemorrhage.

LUNG PROTECTIVE VENTILATION

Permissive Hypercapnia

Permissive hypercapnia is a technique that is used for lung protection during ventilation in order to prevent lung damage and also for patients in the presence of respiratory failure.

Permissive hypercapnia entails the use of low inspiratory pressure and volume while the patient is being ventilated; the greatest concerns with this therapy are the possible development of acidosis, carbon dioxide retention, and hypoventilation.

Recent research indicates that permissive hypercapnia can improve tissue oxygenation, decrease blood lactate levels, increase cardiac output, and the differences between venous oxygen content and arterial oxygen content can be decreased.

Using this approach, the ventilator volumes or pressures should be as low as possible in order to prevent bronchopulmonary dysplasia and barotraumas. An elevated Paco2 is acceptable provided that the pH is 7.25 or more. Similarly, a Pao2 as low as 40 mm Hg is alright if blood pressure is normal and metabolic acidosis is not present.

Optimizing Patient-Ventilator Interaction

The five factors that impact on patient-ventilator interaction are:

1. *Dead space and resistance*
2. *Air leaks*
3. *Compressible volume*
4. *Resistance*
5. *Humidification*

Dead Space and Resistance

Dead space includes the gas volumes contained in the endotracheal tube, the Y connector, monitoring devices attached to the endotracheal connector, the elbow, and the conducing airways, all of which are considered areas of mechanical dead space. All of these gases can be rebreathed. The patient also has anatomical dead space from their airways that are not included in, or affected with, the mechanical dead space of the mechanical ventilation circuit.

Pediatric patients are monitored for the rebreathing of carbon dioxide as a result of this dead space. This aspect of patient-ventilator interaction can be optimized with monitoring and the use of an endotracheal tube that is at the highest possible point of circuit resistance.

Air Leaks

Air leaks which most often occur with a tracheostomy tube or a cuff-less endotracheal tube can adversely affect the tidal volume, ventilator triggering, and lung distending pressures.

The possible presence of air leaks are monitored and detected by comparing the patient's exhaled tidal volume and the ventilator-delivered tidal volume or with the monitoring and review of the patient's ventilator graphics and waveforms

The correction of air leaks may involve re-intubation when changing to higher flow rate and pressure do not deliver an adequate volume.

Compressible Volume

Compressible volume losses must be differentiated from air leaks, particularly among the pediatric population. Compressed gases are delivered from the ventilator but not to the patient. Instead, this compressed volume moves through the exhalation valve and, as such, it adds to the patient's actual exhaled volume. This factor then impacts on the actual volumes delivered to the patient.

Humidification

The purpose of humidification is to reduce the thickness of secretions thus making it easier for the patient to remove them and to prevent any drying from oxygen therapy. The American Association for Respiratory Care established the need for supplemental humidity for all oxygen flows of 4 L/min or more as its standard of practice. Patients with a bypassed upper airway, as is the case among patients with a tracheostomy or endotracheal tube, can be adversely affected with a humidity deficit if adequate heated humidification is not provided.

There are several types of humidifiers including bubble, jet and underwater.

Bubble type humidifiers deliver humidity through a diffusion head or a perforated tube that breaks up the oxygen into small bubbles. This bubble creation facilitates greater surface area contact between the oxygen and the humidity. Bubble type humidifier reservoirs should remain as full as possible; low water levels lower the relative evaporation.

Jet humidifiers create aerosolized droplets. These humidifiers have the ability to deliver moisture at the same relative humidity even when the water level drops, and they can also deliver a higher relative humidity than a bubble type humidifier.

Underwater jet humidifiers provide humidity with an aerosol and water vapor. Of all humidification devices, these humidifiers deliver the highest possible relative humidity. Strict infection control practices must, however, be maintained in order to prevent aerosolized pathogens from entering the respiratory tract. The humidifier and the water must be changed at least every day.

Humidification is used among mechanically ventilated patients in order to prevent complications such as bronchospasm, hypothermia, adverse changes of the airway epithelium, atelectasis, and airway obstruction.

Because the upper airway supplies the alveoli with about 75% of their moisture and heat, humidification is necessary when this upper airway is bypassed. It is suggested that ventilated patients have from a 33 mg H2O/L to a 44 mg H2O/L humidity level and a temperature from 34°C to 41°C with a RH of 100%.

The American National Standards Institute and the American Association for Respiratory Care recommend an absolute humidity of ≥30 mg H2O/L. A temperature of 37 degrees C and a water content of 44 mg is typically adequate.

The two basic methods of humidification are passive humidification with a heat and moisture exchanger, and active humidification using a heated humidifier.

A heat and moisture exchanger (HME), however, when the patient has an expired tidal volume < 70%, copious, thick and bloody secretions, a bodily temperature of <32 °C, and some other alterations. A heat and moisture exchanger is preferred over a heated humidifier during patient transport and for short term use of less than 96 hours.

The complications associated with humidification are an infection and accidental overheating, therefore, humidifiers must be monitored in terms of their temperature and water content and the proper cleaning and disinfection of these devices can prevent infection.

PREVENTING VENTILATOR-ASSOCIATED PNEUMONIA

A number of preventive measures can and should be used to prevent ventilator associated pneumonia, one of the major complications associated with ventilation. Some of these interventions include:

- *Bed position*

- *Cuff pressure*

- *Circuit changes*

- *The proper care of heated humidifiers and heat/ moisture exchangers*

- *Oral care*

- *Secretion removal*

- *Kinetic bed therapy*

- *Sedation reduction*

- *Evaluating weaning readiness and minimizing intubation time*

Bed Position

The head of the bed should be kept at an angle of 30 to 45 degrees unless contraindicated because this angle prevents aspiration.

Cuff Pressure

The cuff pressure should be kept between 20 and 25 cm H2O.

Circuit Change

Circuit changes should not be done routinely, but instead, whenever there is visible soiling.

Heated Humidifiers, and Heat and Moisture Exchangers

The Centers for Disease Control and Prevention (CDC) suggests that heat and moisture exchangers are not changed more than every 48 hours or when they become visibly soiled.

Oral Care

2% chlorhexidine has been found to decrease the risk of ventilator-associated pneumonia.

Secretion Removal with Specially Designed Endotracheal Tubes

The CDC states that when feasible, we should use an endotracheal tube with a dorsal lumen above the endotracheal cuff to allow drainage with continuous or frequent intermittent suctioning of tracheal secretions that accumulate in the patient's subglottic area.

Kinetic Bed Therapy

Evidence suggests that kinetic bed therapy can decrease the risk of lobar atelectasis as well as ventilator-associated pneumonia.

Sedation Reduction

The patient should regularly be tested on their ability to sustain adequate ventilation, oxygenation, and breathing comfort by conducting a spontaneous breathing trial. This can significantly reduce the duration of mechanical ventilation.

Weaning Readiness

Using daily brief weaning trials allow the assessment of the patient's ability to sustain ventilation, oxygenation, breathing comfort, and hemodynamic stability with spontaneous breathing. Combining this with daily sedation assessments has been shown to decrease the duration of mechanical ventilation.

SELECTING, ASSEMBLING AND TROUBLESHOOTING EQUIPMENT

OXYGEN ADMINISTRATION DEVICES

The purpose of oxygen therapy, or oxygen supplementation, is to ensure cellular oxygenation when the patient is adversely affected with one or more acute or chronic respiratory disorders.

The ordered amount of oxygen should be based on the current arterial blood gases or the pulse oximetry reading and the amount of supplemental oxygen should maintain the Pao2 between 60 and 80 mm Hg and 92% to 100% saturation without any signs of oxygen intoxication, or toxicity. The lowest possible Fio2 that maintains an acceptable Pao2 should be given; a Fio2 > 60% is not used except under dire life threatening emergencies. A Fio2 < 40% with a nasal cannula or simple face mask; a Fio2 > 40% requires use of an oxygen mask with an inflated reservoir. Humidification is used with oxygen therapy to moisten secretions and to facilitate easier production.

OXYGEN DELIVERY SYSTEMS

Oxygen systems are categorized as low-flow and high-flow systems. Low-flow devices combine the oxygen with room air and the amount of oxygen delivered is a function of the patient's tidal volume and respiratory rate. High-flow systems, on the other hand, deliver a precise amount of oxygen regardless of the patient's tidal volume or respiratory rate. They include:

- *Low-flow nasal cannulas*

- *Reservoir nasal cannulas*

- *Face masks including the Venturi air entrapment mask*

- *Oxygen hoods*

- *Air entrainment masks*

- *High-flow nasal cannulas*

Low-Flow Nasal Cannulas

A nasal cannula, a low-flow device, is the most commonly used and the least expensive oxygen delivery device that is relatively comfortable and does not interfere with patient activities such as eating and talking. Humidification is provided when the flow is > 4 L/min.

A nasal cannula can be used among cooperative children and adults, however, because they are easily displaced. The nurse must monitor the patient and also use a water soluble gel when the nares become dry.

Reservoir Nasal Cannulas

A reservoir nasal cannula, which is also referred to as Oxidizer, is an oxygen-conserving device. This means that when the patient is breathing out, the reservoir stores oxygen so that when the patient inhales they are able to receive a 100% oxygen bolus. Due to these cannulas' ability to conserve oxygen, they have the ability to provide the patient with higher oxygen concentration at a lower flow rate than the standard nasal cannula.

Face Masks

Face masks that cover a patient's nose and mouth also have ports on the side to allow the carbon dioxide to be released upon exhalation. It is important to make sure that the patient's face is kept dry while using a face mask. Face masks for oxygen therapy are classified as simple, a partial re-breather, a non-breather, and an air entrapment mask.

A simple face mask can deliver a concentration of oxygen between 40 and 60% percent. The partial re-breather mask delivers the same oxygen concentration as the simple face mask, but the simple mask has a liter flow of 5 to 8 L/min and the partial re-breather has a liter flow of 6 to 10 L/min. The oxygen reservoir bag that is attached to the partial re-breather mask allows the patient to rebreathe approximately one-third of the exhaled air mixed with oxygen.

There is also a non-breather mask, which is able to deliver an oxygen concentration of between 95 to 100%. This mask is used with intubation or mechanical ventilation. The room air and the exhaled air are not able to enter the patient because there is a one-way valve that prevents it from doing so.

Finally there is an air entrapment mask called the Venturi mask, which delivers an oxygen concentration of 24 to 50% at a liter flow of 4 to 10 L/min. Its wide bore tubing which allows for high-flow. This mask has different color-coded jet adapters that are used depending on the oxygen concentration and liter flow. For example there can be a blue adapter and a green adapter. The blue adapter can deliver a 35% concentration and 8 L/min; the green adapter can deliver 24% oxygen concentration and 4 L/min. It is important to note that different manufacturers use different color adapters for concentrations, and some use dials or settings to provide different concentrations and/or flow rates.

All face masks should be of proper size and a snug fit which is not tolerated by some patients, particularly pediatric patients, however, since many pediatric patients are mouth breathers, this mask is good for delivery high oxygen flow rates to these patients because the mask, unlike a nasal cannula, covers both the mouth and the nose.

Oxygen Hoods

Oxygen hoods are primarily used for neonates and infants. This plastic hood covers the infant's head and it must deliver at least 5 to 5 L/min to prevent the buildup of carbon dioxide. Additionally, the neck, shoulders or chin should not touch the hood and a pulse oximeter should be used to facilitate continuous SaO2 monitoring and assessments.

High-Flow Nasal Cannulas

High-flow nasal cannulas provide humidified oxygen with a high minute volume when a high FiO2 is necessary to maintain the patient;

prior to the use of these delivery devices, it was necessary to use a special face mask or intubation.

High-flow nasal cannulas are particularly useful for neonates with respiratory distress syndrome in terms of preventing some of the complications of oxygen toxicity such as retinopathy and also in terms of preventing intubation.

COMPLICATIONS OF OXYGEN SUPPLEMENTATION

Some of the complications of oxygen supplementation include:

- *Combustion*
- *Oxygen toxicity*
- *Denitrogenation absorption atelectasis*
- *Retinopathy of prematurity*

Combustion

Oxygen safety in the healthcare setting and the home environment is necessary in order to prevent a fire. For example, "No Smoking" signs should be placed in the home, fibers other than cotton (synthetic fibers) are eliminated because of the risk of static electricity, children's toys that can produce a spark should be avoided, and the use of any flammable liquids like alcohol or acetone near the oxygen source should be discontinued. In the hospital, oxygen tanks must be safely secured and transported.

Oxygen Toxicity

Oxygen toxicity can result from oxygen supplementation therapy when the level of oxygen concentration is too high, when the duration of the therapy is prolonged, and when the severity of lung disease is so severe that higher levels of oxygen concentration are necessary to preserve life.

A loss of consciousness can occur when the PaCO2 is increased and the patient is hypoventilating. Continuous monitoring of the blood gases for oxygen and carbon dioxide levels and maintaining the PaO2 level between 50 and 60 torr can prevent this O2 induced hypoventilation.

Denitrogenation Absorption Atelectasis

Denitrogenation absorption atelectasis can occur when more than 80% oxygen is administered; retinopathy of prematurity, formerly referred to as retrolental fibroplasia, is blindness that some believe can occur. Pulmonary O_2 toxicity can occur among patients who are given more than 50% oxygen for more than 72 hours; CNS abnormalities such as seizures and muscular tremors can occur when a patient is receiving 100% in a hyperbaric chamber.

Some of the greatest risks among infants and young children include hypoventilation, respiratory acidosis, and respiratory arrest when the normal breathing drive is hampered with excessive and chronic carbon dioxide retention as the result of a pulmonary disorder like cystic fibrosis or bronchopulmonary dysplasia. This complication can be prevented with the close monitoring of the Spo2 and the Pao2. The hypoxemia has to be corrected without any compromise in terms of decreasing the pH.

Retinopathy of Prematurity

Although there is still a lot of debate revolving around whether or not the development of retinopathy of prematurity is a complication of oxygen therapy, it appears that this disorder is also the possible result of a number of different factors such as intraventricular hemorrhage, sepsis, a low birth weight, and a premature gestational age. As a result of this possible concern, the oxygen therapy for neonates and infants who weigh less than 1500 g should maintain the Spo2 between 89% and 90% and a Pao2 between 50 and 80 mm Hg.

Other complications of oxygen therapy, in addition to those above, include pulmonary fibrosis and pulmonary vasodilation.

AEROSOL DELIVERY DEVICES

Aerosols can be delivered with nebulizers and in line devices.

NEBULIZERS

There are several types of nebulizers, as below.

- *Air entrainment*
- *Breath activated*
- *Large volume*

- *Ultrasonic*
- *Vibrating mesh*
- *Pressurized metered dose*

Air Entrainment Nebulizers

Air entrainment nebulizers are useful when high levels of humidity and aerosol are indicated. It can be delivered with a face tent, a T piece connected to an endotracheal tube, and a tracheostomy collar which are connected to a corrugated tube and a nebulizer unit.

Breath Activated Nebulizers

Breath activated nebulizers are an alternative to continuous nebulization. It is delivered when the patient's thumb directs the gas delivery only inspiration or with a one-way valve. The aerosol is delivered synchronously with the respiratory cycle, and it can deliver the same and even more of a dosage but it takes about four times longer to deliver the medication.

Large Volume Nebulizers

Large volume nebulizers, with a reservoir that holds more than 100 ml, are indicated when the patient needs prolonged treatment with a solution such as sterile water or a saline solution when the upper airway is bypassed and/or to loosen secretions, induce sputum, and to control stridor.

These devices are not recommended for use in an incubator or hood because the noise produced exceeds the recommended decibel level of 58 decibels as recommended by the American Academy of Pediatrics.

Ultrasonic Nebulizers

Ultrasonic nebulizers can deliver greater aerosol density and a quite broad range of output from 0.5 to 7.0 mL/min. The size of the particles has an inverse relationship to the frequency of the ultrasonic vibrations.

Electrical Vibrating Mesh Nebulizers

Electrical vibrating mesh nebulizers pump medications with the use of a peizo element that vibrates a metal or ceramic disk. The generated particles vary in size according to the size of the openings through which the medication passes without any heating or re-concentration.

Pressurized Metered Dose Inhalers

Pressurized metered dose inhalers are the most commonly used device for aerosolization. They are hand held, and they are simple to use. Some of the medications that can be administered with a pressurized metered dose inhaler include anti-inflammatory, bronchodilating, and anticholinergic drugs.

One of the disadvantages of these inhalers is the fact that the dosage of the medication is dependent upon the patient's proper use of the device; therefore, respiratory therapists must teach patients about their proper use.

NITRIC OXIDE DELIVERY DEVICES

As previously stated, nitric oxide (NO) diffuses through the alveolar membrane to the smooth where it increases the levels of cyclic guanosine monophosphate which, in turn, relaxes them. Nitric oxide therapy is used for respiratory disorders such as:

- *Persistent pulmonary hypertension of the neonate*

- *Chronic obstructive pulmonary disease*

- *Adult respiratory distress syndrome*

The equipment that is used for the delivery of nitric oxide in today's respiratory care environment includes a nitrogen delivery system, a humidifier, a nitric oxide monitor and nitric dioxide monitor.

These devices range in size and there are some specifically made battery ones to facilitate patient transport. As with all respiratory care equipment, the respiratory therapist must ensure that the equipment is safe and in good operating condition. All connections must be checked and all alarms must be set and monitored.

TRANSCUTANEOUS MONITORING SYSTEMS

Transcutaneous oxygen and carbon dioxide levels can be continuously monitored to determine the patient's ability to deliver oxygen to bodily tissues and to remove carbon dioxide during the respiratory cycle.

Transcutaneous electrodes, placed on the skin, measure the gas tension of the underlying tissue rather than a direct measure of arterial gases tension, however, these two measurements closely approximate the PO2 which can be just slightly lower than that in the arteries; the Pco2 is slightly higher.

The electrode is placed on a well vascularized site on the chest, lower arm, back, thigh, or abdomen. Pre-ductal oxygenation levels are obtained when the electrode is placed on the right side of the upper chest; post-ductal oxygenation levels are obtained when the electrode is placed on the left side of the upper chest. The sensor heat level is typically between 43 and 44 degrees C but those with thicker skin require a slightly higher temperature.

There are now newer noninvasive methods that combine transcutaneous carbon dioxide measurements with arterial oxygen saturation using a sensor heated to about 42c degrees C that is placed on the ear.

MECHANICAL VENTILATORS

Respiratory therapists must refer to the facility's policies and procedures as well as the mechanical ventilator's manufacturer instructions on setting up and troubleshooting mechanical ventilators. Some of the basic guidelines for setting up and troubleshooting mechanical ventilators include ensuring that:

- All connections and hoses are tight and secure

- The power source such as the electrical outlet is operable

- All filters are free of debris and they are intact

- Gas connections are safe, stable, secure, and in good operating condition

- There is no obstruction from plugging and excessive secretions

- Water levels are maintained

Newer and more advanced mechanical ventilators have self-diagnostic capabilities.

MECHANICAL INSUFFLATION-EXSUFFLATION

Mechanical insufflation-exsufflation devices are used to promote the patient's cough in order to clear the respiratory airway of secretions, as is often necessary among patients affected with a muscular, pulmonary and/or CNS disorder which prevents effective coughing.

Mechanical insufflation-exsufflation therapy, with a device such as the CoughAssist In-Exsufflator gradually insufflates, or inflates, the lungs after which there is a rapid change to negative pressure which produces rapid exsufflation, or exhalation. After these rapid insufflation-exsufflation cycles, the cough is stimulated and the secretions are removed and loosened.

The setup is quite simple. Tubing and a mask is used to connect the patient to the device. Also, these devices can be used in the home after patient/family education and training.

An alternative to insufflation-exsufflation is insufflation to maximum insufflation capacity using breath-stacking with a bag and mask, a volume ventilator, or glossopharyngeal breathing.

HIGH FREQUENCY CHEST OSCILLATION

High frequency chest wall oscillation effectively increases the clearance of tracheal mucous using a vest like device that is worn by the patient. When this un-stretchable vest is connected to the air pulse generator, it deflates and inflates on the patient's chest about 5 to 20 times a second and, with this rapid action, it facilitates the patient's cough which enables the dislodgment of retained secretions.

PERFORMING AND ASSISTING WITH PROCEDURES

Some of the special procedures that respiratory therapists participate in include:

- *Inter- or Intra-hospital transport*

- *Intravascular catheter insertion*

- *Bronchoscopy and associated procedures*

- *Intubation*

- *Extubation*

INTERHOSPITAL AND INTRA HOSPITAL TRANSPORT

INTERHOSPITAL TRANSPORT

Interhospital transport is highly complex and it often requires the close collaboration of a number of specialized healthcare team members including nurses, respiratory therapists, physicians, emergency medical staff, and a pilot with air transport or a driver for ground transport.

Although requirements may vary a little among the states, the minimum requirements for a transport respiratory therapists includes registration with the National Board for Respiratory Care, state licensure, two years of PICU or NICU experience, the successful completion of a pediatric transport course, the observation of several transports, and current NRP, PALS and BCLS certifications.

The modes of transportation include ground transport and air transport using a rotor wing or fixed wing aircraft such as a helicopter and a jet, respectively. Both modes of transport have advantages and disadvantages.

Some of the advantages of ground transportation, when compared to air transport, include its lower cost, its ability to transport with inclement weather, its capabilities for going from one medical center to another, and fewer numbers of staff. A primary disadvantage of ground transportation is its relative lack of speed when compared to air transport, particularly when there is traffic congestion.

Some of the advantages of air transport include its ability to travel for long distances and its speed, which can be as much as or more than 120 miles per hour. Its disadvantages include its relatively high cost and the need to have an ambulance at the beginning and end of the flight transport unless the facilities have helicopter pads and/or landing and takeoff fields.

Some of the physiological concerns relating to air transportation include the principles of Boyle's and Dalton's law.

Boyle's law states that volume is inversely proportionate to pressure. When the temperature in the helicopter or fixed wing plane remains constant at the same time that the altitude of the plane increases, the volume of gases within the plane expand. The infant or young child may, therefore, be affected with nausea, vomiting, increased pain, increase respiratory depth and rate, changes in the intravenous flow rates, and endotracheal tube cuff expansion.

Dalton's law states that the pressure of gas mixtures is equal to the sum of the partial pressures of the gases that make up the mixture of gases. As a result of this law of physics, the patient will have a reduced delivery of oxygen because of the decrease in partial pressure as the aircraft climbs and the barometric pressure decreases at the same time that the fraction of the inspired oxygen remains constant at 21%.

Both modes of transport need communication systems, monitoring equipment such as an ECG, pulse oximeter, blood pressure equipment, and methods to assess the patient's bodily temperature as well as a wide variety of other medical equipment such as:

- *A mechanical ventilator*

- *A transport incubator for infants less 5 kg of body weight*

- *Infusion pumps and devices*

- *Point of care testing equipment and supplies*

- *Medications*

- *Medical gases*

INTRAHOSPITAL TRANSPORT

Intrahospital transport, or the movement of the patient from one area of the hospital to another is, for obvious reasons, far less complicated and challenging than ground and air transport to another facility, however, this type of transport also requires patient stabilization, communication, and collaboration.

INTRAVASCULAR CATHETER INSERTION

Respiratory therapists often assist with the insertion of intravascular catheters, such as venous and arterial catheters as well as drawing samples from these lines or catheters.

Arterial catheters include:

- *Peripheral artery catheters*

- *Umbilical artery catheters*

- *Pulmonary artery catheters*

Venous catheters include:

- *Central venous catheters*

- *Peripheral venous catheters*

PERIPHERAL ARTERY CATHETERS

Peripheral artery catheters are used for pediatric patients to monitor blood gases. These catheters can be placed through the skin using the percutaneous method or with a cut down which is a small surgical incision that permits direct visualization of the vessels.

The most commonly used site is the radial artery; however, other arteries such as the dorsalis pedis, the posterior tibial, the brachial, the femoral, or the brachial arteries can be used.

A transillumination light may be useful for the location of the artery among infants and young children.

UMBILICAL ARTERY CATHETERS

Neonates have two accessible arteries in the umbilicus immediately after delivery. The two positions of the umbilical artery catheter are the high position and the low position. The complications of both positions include hypotension, hypoglycemia, vasospasm, and possible emboli distal to the catheter tip.

The length of the catheter that will be used is based on the distance from the umbilicus to the shoulder which is then used as a reference post on a nomogram which indicates the correct catheter insertion distance.

The catheter placement and patency are confirmed after which it is connected to a fluid pressure transducer.

PULMONARY ARTERY CATHETERS

Pulmonary artery catheters, also referred to as Swan-Ganz catheters, are useful for patients with respiratory failure patients and others who are critically ill. They are useful for monitoring and assessing fluid needs, left ventricular function, cardiovascular monitoring, and pulmonary function. Specifically, they measure pulmonary and cardiac pressures and cardiac output as well as other measurements. They are used more frequently among adults rather than pediatric patients.

Pulmonary artery catheters have four lumens or ports, a balloon, a thermistor, and a thermistor connector. They come in sizes from 5 French for patients less than 18 kg and up to 7 French outer diameters. The four ports and their uses are:

1. *The proximal port: This port is in the right atrium and it measures right atrial pressure.*

2. *The distal port: This lumen lies in the pulmonary artery and it measures pulmonary capillary wedge pressure and pulmonary artery pressure. It is also used to sample mixed venous blood for analysis.*

3. *The inflation port: This port is at the tip of the catheter. When the balloon is inflated correctly it surrounds the tip of the catheter but it does not cover it.*

4. *The temperature measuring thermistor port: This port connects the catheter to the cardiac output monitor.*

The patient is placed in the Trendelenburg position to increase neck vein filling and to prevent air embolism for placement. The pulmonary artery catheter is then inserted percutaneously, or with a cut-down, and then advanced until the right atrial pressure waveform is seen on the monitor. Later, the balloon is inflated and moved into the right ventricle through the mitral valve. Lastly, the catheter is then advanced into the pulmonary artery and wedged so the catheter occludes the artery after which the balloon is deflated when proper placement is confirmed with waveforms.

Some of the complications associated with pulmonary artery catheters include hemorrhage, thrombosis, sepsis, arrhythmias, pneumothorax, pulmonic valve damage, tricuspid valve damage, right ventricular perforation, and right atrial perforation.

CENTRAL VENOUS CATHETERS

Central venous catheters are indicated for a number of conditions including:

- *The lack of an adequate peripheral access site*

- *The need to administer fluids, medications, and/or parenteral nutrition*

- *Significant cardiovascular instability*

- *Volume disturbances such as hemorrhage, increased intracranial pressure, and extreme dehydration*

- *The necessity of monitoring the patient's central venous pressure*

The insertion techniques for the insertion of a central venous catheter varies according to the age and the physical status of the child or infant. Like other catheters, these lines can be placed with a percutaneous stick or with a surgical cut down. The most commonly used vessels for the percutaneous method of insertion are the internal and external jugular veins, the brachial vein, the saphenous veins, and the subclavian vein.

These catheters are inserted using sterile technique. The patient is typically sedated and the site is anesthetized with a topical agent like lidocaine. The placement is confirmed when the right atrial pressure waveform appears and with x-rays. After this confirmation, the catheter is connected to a flush line and pressure transducer.

Among the several complications of central venous lines are sepsis and pulmonary embolism.

PERIPHERAL VENOUS CATHETERS

Peripheral venous catheters are used primarily for fluid management, electrolyte replacement, and medication administration.

Peripheral venous catheters are classified as peripheral catheters, midline peripheral catheters, and peripherally inserted central catheters.

Although respiratory therapists do not insert, maintain, or use peripheral venous catheters, except under rare circumstances, respiratory therapists should be aware of their complications because many of these complications impact on the patient's cardiopulmonary status.

Some of these complications include:

- *Infection*
- *Infiltration*
- *Extravasation*

- *Phlebitis*
- *Occlusions*
- *Embolus*

BRONCHOSCOPY AND ASSOCIATED PROCEDURES

BRONCHOSCOPY

Diagnostic bronchoscopy is done to assess and diagnose a number of pulmonary disorders when a less invasive method is not appropriate and therapeutic bronchoscopy is done for treatments.

Diagnostic bronchoscopy is used when the airway anatomy has to be determined, for inhalation injury evaluation, hemoptysis evaluation, to diagnose functional airway problems like vocal cord dysfunction and bronchomalacia, as well as when there has been a possible foreign body aspiration.

Flexible fiber optic bronchoscopes, rather than rigid bronchoscopes, are used unless wider channels are needed such as when an aspirated foreign body has to be removed.

In addition to diagnostic bronchoscopy, which directly visualizes the airway up to and including the sub-segmental bronchi, bronchoscopy also permits treatments and diagnostic interventions such as laser therapy, removing a foreign body, medication administration with drugs such as N acetyl cysteine, endotracheal intubation, suctioning, taking a biopsy, and sampling of respiratory secretions.

Prior to bronchoscopy, the necessary and possibly necessary supplies and equipment should be collected for ready access. Some of these items include the bronchoscope with a light source, an endotracheal tube swivel adapter, monitoring equipment like a respiratory monitor, pulse oximeter and cardiac monitor, oxygen and aerosol supplies like oxygen delivery devices, an oxygen source and necessary tubing, specimen collection equipment like a Luken trap, a channel brush and a biopsy forceps, suction equipment and supplies like a vacuum source, suction catheters including a Yankauer catheter and a tonsil tip catheter, topical anesthetics like lidocaine, sedatives like diazepam and midazolam, and intravenous equipment and supplies.

Most pediatric patients, and adults as well, need some sedation when they are having a bronchoscopy done. This sedation can be administered intramuscularly or intravenously. The preferred route is intravenously because it has a shorter duration, faster onset, and it can be titrated for desired effects.

The most common form of sedation that is used is conscious sedation using a medication such as a combination of a benzodiazepine and a narcotic like midazolam and fentanyl, respectively.

The usual pediatric dosage of intravenous midazolam is from 0.05 mg/kg to 0.3 mg/kg with a maximum dosage of 0.4 to 0.6 mg/kg. The typical pediatric dosage of fentanyl is 1 ug/kg to 3 ug/kg, which is also titrated according to response, with a maximum dosage of no more than 5 to 10 ug/kg.

Other conscious sedation medications that are used include intramuscular chlorpromazine, promethazine, and meperidine and a combination of droperidol, thorazine and promethazine. Lastly, nasally inhaled midazolam can also be used.

The vocal cords and pharynx are anesthetized with aerosol or nebulized lidocaine. The bronchoscope is then lubricated and passed through the airway and past the vocal cords into the bronchi during inspiration.

BRONCHOALVEOLAR LAVAGE (BAL)

Bronchoalveolar lavage (BAL) is a diagnostic procedure which entails the passing of a bronchoscopy tube into the lung, after which a fluid is instilled into the lung and then collected for analysis. It is of limited value in terms of diagnosing lung diseases and disorders because the range of normal values is rather large. Despite its limitations, bronchoalveolar lavage is sometimes done to aid in the diagnosis of alveolar hemorrhage, pneumonia, other infections, malignancies, and alveolar and/or interstitial infiltrates.

BIOPSIES

In addition to diagnostic bronchoscopy which directly visualizes the airway up to and including the sub-segmental bronchi, bronchoscopy also enables taking a biopsy of suspicious tissue.

A sample of the tissue is taken using a biopsy forceps after which it is sent to a laboratory for pathology.

BRUSHING

Brushing is another technique that is used to obtain a biopsy. This procedure uses a brush rather than a forceps to obtain the tissue sample. This technique is also used for the detection of oral cancer and for removing tissue from the lining of the ureter or kidney.

EXTUBATION

Weaning, weaning readiness and weaning methods were discussed above. Here, there will be a discussion about extubating the patient after the weaning process. The two types of extubation are accidental extubation and planned extubation.

ACCIDENTAL EXTUBATION

The risk factors associated with accidental extubations among the neonatal and pediatric populations include insufficient sedation, a failure to secure the tube adequately, the lack of ordered restraints to prevent self extubation, and accidents that occur during a medical or diagnostic procedure.

In contrast, the risk factors associated with accidental extubation among adults is self extubation despite the fact that the patient is sedated and restrained. Fortunately, accidental extubations are rare and when they do occur, they usually do not lead to mortality.

The treatment for accidental extubations include the reinsertion of the tube if the need for it is present.

PLANNED EXTUBATION

Planned extubation occurs after successful weaning and respiratory stability. This procedure entails:

- *Suctioning of the trachea and oropharynx*
- *The administration of a B agonist*
- *Discontinuing any enteral feedings if used*
- *Cuff deflation*
- *Removing tape and other securing devices*
- *The patient's taking or receiving one deep breath*
- *Rapidly removing the tube*
- *Administering oxygen as needed*

DELIVERING PHARMACOLOGICAL AGENTS

BASIC MEDICATION TERMS AND DEFINITIONS

Chemical name: The chemical composition of the drug.

Trade or brand name: The manufacturer's name for the drug. Trade name drugs are more expensive than generic drugs.

Generic name: The name of a drug that can include a number of different trade names. For example, metoprolol, which is a generic name, can have equivalent trade names such as Lopressor and Metoprolol Succinate ER.

Drug absorption: Absorption occurs as the medication moves through the digestive tract. Rates of absorption vary according to the acidity of the stomach's fluids and the presence of food, for example.

Drug distribution: After absorption, the components of the medication move in the bloodstream to the intended target.

Drug metabolism or biotransformation: The breakdown of a drug, or medication, in the liver.

Excretion: Most drugs are excreted through the kidney, but some are also excreted with feces and respiratory expiration.

Therapeutic or desired effect: A therapeutic effect is the primary, expected effect of a specific medication. For example, the therapeutic effect of metoprolol is to lower blood pressure.

Side effects: A side effect of a medication is a secondary, not primary, effect of a medication. Side effects are either minor or major, and are either desirable or detrimental.

Idiosyncratic effects: Unexpected side effects that are peculiar and specific to a particular patient. When a sedative makes a person agitated, rather than sedated, this is an idiosyncratic effect.

Cumulative effects: The buildup of medication in the patient's system as a result of impaired excretion or metabolism of the drug, which can lead to toxic effects.

Adverse effects: The most serious side effects of drugs that lead to the immediate discontinuation of the medication. Adverse effects must be reported.

Drug toxicity: An over dosage of a medication that occurs when the patient's metabolism and/or excretion is impaired.

Potentiating effect: A synergistic effect results from the combination of two or more drugs where the effects of one, or both, are increased.

Inhibiting effect: An inhibiting effect is one that results from the combination of two or more drugs where the effects of one, or both, are decreased.

Drug allergy: An antigen- antibody immunologic response to a medication. All patients must be assessed for any drug sensitivities or allergies.

Anaphylactic reaction: The most severe of all medication allergy response which can be life threatening. The throat and tongue swell, obstructing the airway.

Drug tolerance: This often occurs when a patient has been receiving an opioid for an extended period of time. The patient needs increasing doses of the drug in order to achieve the therapeutic effect.

Drug interaction: Drugs can interact with a number of things including other prescribed drugs, over-the-counter medications, foods, herbs, supplements, and other natural substances.

ROUTES OF MEDICATION ADMINISTRATION

The oral route is the preferred route of administration for all patients whenever possible; however it is contraindicated for a patient who is affected with a swallowing disorder and/or unconsciousness, for example.

Age-Specific Considerations

- *Infants*

Dosages are based on kilograms of weight and/or body surface area.

- *Toddlers*

Dosages continue to be based on kilograms of weight.

- *Preschool and school age children*

Dosages are based on kilograms of weight.

- *Adolescents*

Adult dosages, routes and forms of medications are indicated and acceptable.

- *The elderly*

Dosages may be decreased among the elderly because the normal physiological changes of the aging process make them more susceptible to side effects, adverse drug reactions, toxicity and over dosage.

The renal function among the elderly is affected with diminished blood flow, reduced creatinine clearance, decreased drug clearance, lower renal mass and decreased glomerular and tubular functioning. Hepatic function is also altered as the result of the normal aging process. Decreased hepatic blood flow, which results in reduced hepatic metabolism and increased concentrations of medications, as well as a smaller hepatic mass, impact on the medications that this population takes.

It is therefore recommended that the lowest possible dose is used initially and then increased slowly over time until the therapeutic effect is achieved. Often, the initial dosage can be only 50% of the recommended adult dosage. Additionally, the elderly patient must be assessed and reassessed for side effects, adverse drug reactions, toxicity and therapeutic effects.

MEDICATION SAFETY

All medications have intended uses, or indications, for use. Some medications are contraindicated for certain patients. For example, a medication can be contraindicated for patients who have an allergy to the medication, hepatic disease and/or renal disease as well as lactating and pregnant women. Other medications may be permitted with caution, or precautions, under certain circumstances. For example, a medication may be used with caution among the elderly population or those with renal disease.

Medications can interact with a number of things. Some interactions include those with other medications including over-the-counter drugs, foods, and lifestyle choices, such as alcohol use, herbs and other natural substances.

Virtually all medications have side effects. Nausea and vomiting are the most common side effects; most side effects are simply troublesome but others, referred to as adverse effects, can be life threatening. There are still more medications are associated with toxic effects. For example, tinnitus is a sign of toxicity associated with aspirin and bradycardia is associated with digitalis toxicity.

THE TEN RIGHTS OF MEDICATION ADMINISTRATION

The "Ten Rights of Medication Administration" are the right, or correct:

1. Medication   *6. Patient education*

2. Dosage   *7. Documentation*

3. Time   *8. Right to refuse*

4. Route   *9. Assessment*

5. Patient   *10. Evaluation*

PATIENTS AT RISK FOR MEDICATION ERRORS

Some groups of patients are more at risk for medication errors than others. Some of the patient populations that are at greatest risk are infants, children, the elderly as well as members of a population that has a language barrier, cognitive impairment, decreased level of consciousness, sensory disorder and/or developmental or psychiatric disorder.

- *Language barriers*

  Individuals with language barriers may not be able to understand you and you may not be able to understand them. Using interpreters, whether they be family or friends, or pictures and drawings, should be utilized to overcome any language barrier.

- *Decreased level of consciousness*

  Medication errors and other mistakes are more likely to occur with patients who are not alert, awake or oriented to time, place and person. Patient identification is critical when providing care to a person with a reduced level of consciousness.

  At times, a visiting family member or friend can assist with patient identification, and can also ask about questionable medications and whether the patient has legally agreed to these types of discussions.

- *Sensory disorders*

  Auditory or visual impairments can lead to medication errors. Eyeglasses, hearing aids, or other assistive devices, must be consistently provided and used by the sensory impaired person to protect their safety.

  If the individual has an auditory impairement, facing the person while speaking and using large print or Braille materials for the visually impaired may offer some protection against medication errors.

- *Cognitive impairments*

  Patients who are demented, confused, disoriented, and/or affected with delirium are at risk for all types of errors. Patient identification is, again, vitally critical. It is also helpful to communicate with the affected person in a way they can understand and to listen to, and observe their nonverbal communication, carefully. The respiratory therapist should also encourage the active participation of the significant other(s) and use drawings and pictures to facilitate communicate.

- *Developmental and psychiatric disorders*

  Lastly, patients with a psychiatric or developmental disorder are at risk for medication errors, some of which can be very serious. For example, many psychotropic medications have sedating effects, therefore posing the same safety challenges as those with reduced levels of consciousness. This population may also be delusional and out of touch with reality.

  Accurate identification is necessary during all aspects of care, especially during medication administration. At least two (2) unique identifiers, other than room number, must be used. Some examples of unique identifiers include a unique code number, the person's first, middle and last name and/or complete date of birth including year, an encoded bar code with at least 2 unique identifiers imbedded into it and a photograph.

MEDICATION DOCUMENTATION

Complete and acceptable medication administration records must minimally include the patient's full name, room and bed number for inpatients, age, physician name, any allergies, name of the ordered medication(s), dosage, route and form of the medication, date and time that the order was written, date(s) and time(s) of administration, start and end dates of the order, the initials and signatures, and the title(s), such as CRT, of all those who have administered the medication(s.)

A medication that is administered, omitted, held or refused by the patient must be documented in the patient's medication record and/or progress note, according to the facility's specific policy and procedure.

Calculating Dosages

The three systems of measurement used in pharmacology are the household measurement system, the metric system and the apothecary system. Each system can be converted to another system when the proper equivalents are used for this mathematical calculation. The ten most commonly used equivalents are:

- *1 Kg = 1,000 g*

- *1 Kg = 2.2 lbs.*

- *1 L = 1,000 mL*

- *1 g = 1,000 mg*

- *1 mg = 1,000 mcg*

- *1 gr = 60 mg*

- *1 oz. = 30 g or 30 mL*

- *1 tsp. = 5 mL*

- *1 lb. = 454 g*

- *1 Tbsp. = 15 mL*

Pediatric Dosages

Pediatric dosages are based on body weight and body surface area.

RESPIRATORY MEDICATION

RESPIRATORY MEDICATION ADMINISTRATION ROUTES

Respiratory therapists use medications that are administered in different forms and routes. Some of these include:

- *Aerosolized medications*

- *Dry powder preparations*

- *Medications administered via an endotracheal tube*

Simply defined, an aerosolized and/or nebulized medication is one that contains small particles of a medication that can be dispensed directly into the respiratory tract. The most commonly used nebulized aerosol medications are mucolytic drugs, bronchodilators, corticosteroids and antibiotics.

COMMONLY USED RESPIRATORY CARE MEDICATIONS

Respiratory therapists must be fully knowledgeable about all the medications that they administer, and also some of the medications that others administer which might impact on the patient's cardiopulmonary status. They must be cognitively competent in terms of these medications, their indications, contraindications, actions, side effects, adverse reactions and dosages. Some of the medications that the respiratory therapist must know about include:

- *Antibiotics*
- *Mucolytic drugs*
- *Leukotriene Modifiers*
- *Bronchodilators*

- *Anti-inflammatory corticosteroids*
- *Vasodilators*
- *Mast cell stabilizers*

Antibiotics or Antimicrobials

The use of antimicrobials for the treatment of infections is the most common therapeutic treatment. To the greatest extent possible, the selection of the antimicrobial and the dosage should be driven by the specific microorganism and the current physical condition of the host.

Antimicrobial prophylaxis can be a primary prevention or a secondary prevention measure. It is considered primary prevention when it prevents any infection; and it is considered secondary prevention when it treats and prevents the recurrence of an infection.

Antimicrobial prophylaxis is often, and perhaps too often, used to prevent the onset of an infectious disease. For example, preventive prophylactic antibiotics can be used for the prevention of urinary tract infections when a patient has an indwelling urinary catheter, and to prevent other infections such as rheumatic fever which can lead to serious cardiac damage, herpes simplex recurring bouts of cellulitis, meningitis, endocarditis, as well as open wounds and open fracture infections.

Prophylactic antimicrobials, particularly antibacterial drugs, are also used and indicated perioperatively for certain types of surgery, like gastrointestinal and total joint replacement surgical procedures, to prevent surgically related infections. For example, an intravenous antibiotic may be administered ½ hour to 1 hour prior to a surgical procedure.

Ideally, prophylactic antimicrobials should not be used; however, when it is necessary to use them they must be used judiciously. The ideal prophylactic antimicrobial should be limited in terms of the duration of use, inexpensive, nontoxic, target specific and bactericidal. Resistance remains a high public health concern.

The therapeutic use of antimicrobials should, under ideal circumstances, be based on the components of the cycle of infection. For example, it should be based on the site of the infection, the host, and whenever possible, based on a definitive diagnosis of the infection and the offending pathogen. At times, when there is not yet a definitive diagnosis, the empiric use of antimicrobials is indicated.

The identification of the specific offending pathogen is extremely important especially when an infection can be life threatening, when the patient is not responding to current therapeutic interventions and when the course of antimicrobial therapy is anticipated to be rather prolonged.

This identification is dependent upon accurate and timely microbiological laboratory testing prior to the initiation of the therapy, whenever possible. In addition to laboratory testing, the patient's past medical history, including an exposure history, and the presenting signs and symptoms also serve as considerations in terms of exactly which antimicrobial is the most effective and the most appropriate for the patient.

The initiation of the antimicrobial therapy is based on a number of considerations including the condition of the patient. For example, critically ill patients, like those with sepsis, should have an immediate initiation of antimicrobial therapy after diagnostic specimens are obtained. When the patient condition is stable, it is recommended that antimicrobial therapy be postponed until laboratory findings are complete.

The empiric use of antimicrobials is defined as the use of antimicrobial medications based on signs and symptoms in the patient's physical condition, because microbiological results typically take 24 to 72 hours. The antimicrobial agents that are used with empiric diagnoses are typically broad scope agents or a combination of agents until a definitive diagnosis is done.

Other commonly used blood laboratory tests used for infections include the erythrocyte sedimentation rate (ESR), C-reactive protein (CRP) plasma viscosity (PV), all of which are sensitive to increases in protein, which is a part of the inflammation process. The ESR, CRP and PV can be raised with primarily bacterial infections, abscesses and other disorders such as cancer, burns and a myocardial infarction. Some health problems like polycythemia, sickle cell anemia and heart failure can be signaled with a less than normal ESR. Additionally, urine testing and spinal fluid analysis can also be done.

Mucolytic Medications

Mucolytic medications, also referred to as proteolytics, were more often used in the past than they are today.

- *Actions*

  Mucolytic medications loosen and decrease the viscosity of mucus and mucus plugs.

- *Examples*

  Some examples of these medications include acetyl cysteine, RhDNAse, dornase alpha, hypertonic saline and other solutions such as hypotonic saline and normal saline which can be administered with direct instillation into the airway and with an aerosol.

- *Indications*

  These medications are used to treat bronchitis, cystic fibrosis and to induce secretion mobilization and to produce sputum.

Leukotriene Modifiers

Leukotriene modifiers are a separate and newer classification of respiratory medications only given by the oral route.

- *Actions*

  Leukotriene modifiers decrease and suppress bronchoconstriction, airway edema, mucus production and inflammation by preventing the effects of leukotriene.

- *Examples*

  Some examples of leukotriene modifiers are montelukast, sileuton and zafirlukast.

- *Indications*

  These medications are used for adults and children over 15 years of age for the long term treatment of asthma, to decrease episodes of allergic rhinitis and to prevent bronchospasm secondary to exercise.

- *Contraindications and Precautions*

  These medications are contraindicated among children less than 15 years of age and they are used cautiously among patients affected with liver disease and patients who are taking warfarin and theophylline.

- *Side Effects and Adverse Reactions*

  Some of the side effects of leukotriene modifiers include liver damage, the inhibition of warfarin metabolism and the inhibition of theophylline which can lead to increased warfarin and theophylline levels, respectively.

Bronchodilators

The pharmacological classification of bronchodilators is also referred to as adrenergic sympathomimetic medications, beta agonists, catecholamines and beta adrenergic agonist medications.

- *Actions*

All bronchodilators stimulate the body's sympathetic nervous system which in turn results in bronchodilation. Bronchodilators also increase ciliary motility and they inhibit the release of histamine.

- *Examples*

Bronchodilators can be classified as ultra-short acting, short acting, intermediate acting and long term acting. Some examples of ultra-short acting bronchodilators are racemic, isoetharine and epinephrine; metaproterenol, pirbutrol and trabutaline are examples of short acting bronchodilators; examples of intermediate acting bronchodilators are levalbuterol and albuterol; formoterol, salmeterol and arformoterol are examples of long acting bronchodilators.

- *Indications*

This classification of medication is indicated for the treatment of asthma, bronchospasm with severe and moderate shortness of breath, laryngeal edema and bleeding/trauma secondary to a bronchoscopy and anaphylaxis. In summary, short acting bronchodilators are used for acute bronchospasms, long duration bronchodilators are used for stable and chronic bronchospasm, and vaso-constricting bronchodilators like epinephrine are used to treat airway bleeding and edema.

- *Contraindications and Precautions*

These medications are Pregnancy Risk Category C; they are used with caution among patients affected with angina, hyperthyroidism, hypertension and diabetes and they are contraindicated when a patient has a cardiac tachydysrhythmia.

- *Side Effects and Adverse Reactions*

Inhaled agents have few side effects and adverse effects; oral bronchodilators can lead to angina, tachycardia, tremors, palpitations, headache, increased blood pressure, dizziness, nausea, irritability, nervousness and decreasing PaO2 as a result of a deteriorating ventilation perfusion ratio.

Anti-Inflammatory Drugs

Anti-inflammatory drugs can be classified in a number of different categories. Some of these categories include:

- *Non-steroidal Anti-Inflamma-tory Drugs (NSAIDS)*
- *Glucocorticoids*

Non-steroidal anti-inflammatory drugs, primarily oral and "over the counter", are used for mild to moderate pain with and without a narcotic analgesic, to decrease inflammation and to treat a fever. Some of the commonly used NSAIDS are acetaminophen, aspirin and aspirin. For the purpose of this discussion, the corticosteroids will be covered in the context of respiratory care.

- *Actions*

Inhaled corticosteroids can be delivered to the patient with a number of different modes and mechanisms. These medications not only halt the inflammatory process in the airways, but also potentiate, or strengthen, the effects of bronchodilating sympathomimetic medications and decrease the production of mucus in the airways.

At times, corticosteroids are also taken orally and intravenously. For example, a patient with status asthmaticus may be given emergency corticosteroids intravenously to reverse this life threatening condition.

Examples of oral glucocorticoids are prednisone and prednisolone; examples of intravenous glucocorticoids are methylprednisolone sodium succinate (Solu-Medrol) and hydrocortisone sodium succinate (Solu-Cortef.)

- *Examples*

Examples of inhaled glucocorticoids are beclomethasone (QVAR), budesonide, budesonide and formoterol, flunisolide hemihydrates HFA, fluticasone propionate, fluticasone propionate and salmeterol, mometasone furoate and triamcinolone acetonide. All of these medications, with the exception of beclomethasone, are taken using a spacer. These medications are not short acting so they do not provide immediate results but they are useful for the prevention of attacks and to decrease the severity of the attack if and when it occurs.

Patients who take both an inhaled glucocorticoid and an inhaled beta adrenergic agonist must be advised to take the beta adrenergic agonist before taking the inhaled glucocorticoid because the former promotes bronchodilation, thus enabling the desired enhancement of the inhaled glucocorticoid.

- *Indications*

These inhaled medications are used to prevent asthma attacks and for the treatment of chronic asthma.

- *Contraindications and Precautions*

These medications are Pregnancy Risk Category C; they are used with caution among the pediatric population, those taking NSAIDS, and among patients affected with renal dysfunction, diabetes, hypertension and/or a peptic ulcer. These medications are contraindicated when the patient is affected with a systemic fungal infection or the patient has recently received a vaccination with a live virus.

- *Side Effects and Adverse Reactions*

The primary side effect of an inhaled glucocorticoid is oral/throat changes such as difficulty speaking, hoarseness and the development of candidiasis.

Vasodilators

Vasodilators are frequently used for the treatment and postoperative care of patients with heart failure.

- *Actions*

Each of the vasodilator categories acts in different ways, however, all have an antihypertensive effect.

- *Examples*

Examples of vasodilators include angiotensin converting enzyme inhibitors like captopril, angiotensin II Receptor blockers like losarten, calcium channel blockers like nifedipine and amlodipine, alpha adrenergic blockers such as doxazosin, centrally acting alpha 2 agonists like clonidine and beta adrenergic blockers such as metoprolol and atenolol.

- *Indications*

Although the vast majority of antihypertensive vasodilators are used among the adult population, children and infants with heart failure are also treated with these medications.

Nitroprusside, for example, is often used for postoperative cardiac surgery hypertension. The dosage of this medication initially is 0.3 to 0.5 mcg/kg/min and then it is titrated to achieve the desired effect. The maintenance dose is typically about 3 mcg/kg/min.

ACE inhibitors like captopril in a dosage of 0.1 to 0.3 mg/kg po tid and β-blockers like carvedilol and metoprolol are also used to treat heart failure among members of the pediatric population.

- *Contraindications and Precautions*

The contraindications and precautions relating to these medications vary according to the classification of the medication.

- *Side Effects and Adverse Reactions*

   Some of the side effects of leukotriene modifiers include liver damage, the inhibition of warfarin metabolism and the inhibition of theophylline, which can lead to increased warfarin and theophylline levels, respectively.

   The primary side effects for these medications are cardiac arrhythmias and hypotension.

Mast Cell Stabilizers

- *Actions*

   Mast cell stabilizers are anti-inflammatory medications that inhibit the release of histamine and other mediators associated with the inflammatory process. They also suppress inflammatory cells like the macrophages and eosinophils by stabilizing the mast cells.

- *Examples*

   Cromolyn sodium is a mast cell stabilizer.

- *Indications*

   Cromolyn sodium is used for the treatment of chronic asthma and the prevention of exercise induced asthma and bronchospasm, allergic rhinitis and allergen induced reactions.

- *Contraindications and Precautions*

   Mast cell stabilizers are Pregnancy Risk Category B; they should be used with caution among patients affected with a kidney or liver disorders as well as among patients with cardiac arrhythmias, coronary artery disease and status asthmaticus.

Respiratory therapists are most often involved in the administration of two airway medications that are instilled; they are surfactant and lidocaine.

Surfactant Replacement Therapy

Surfactant is administered as prophylaxis, and also administered for a number of disorders and diseases such altered surfactant composition, altered surfactant metabolism, altered surfactant quantity, surfactant inactivation, and respiratory distress syndrome. It can be administered as a rescue dose and also as part of a planned treatment.

Exogenous surfactant can be natural or synthetic. Natural surfactant products are derived from primarily bovine and porcine lungs. Some synthetic surfactant products contain protein equivalents and others do not.

Most infants improve with surfactant therapy, but there are some who do not respond. These non-responders are often affected with comorbidities such as congenital heart disease, pulmonary hypoplasia and pneumonia, for example.

Surfactant is delivered by the intra-tracheal route using an endotracheal tube with a side adapter or a Y adapter that is attached to the endotracheal tube. There is no demonstrated need to routinely position or reposition the infant because surfactant has a great capacity to spread; however, some experts recommend repositioning during its administration, so use your professional judgment.

Some of the side effects associated with surfactant are bradycardia, cyanosis, regurgitation of the surfactant into the endotracheal tube and airway obstruction. When these side effects occur, the administration of the surfactant is temporarily halted until the vital signs and the patient are stable. Repositioning the patient into a prone position, increasing the positive pressure ventilation and lowering the bolus dose of the surfactant may correct the problem.

Lidocaine

Lidocaine, with different routes of administration, has several uses and indications for those with cardiopulmonary disorders. Examples are as follows:

- *Intravenous lidocaine* is used for the treatment of severe cardiac arrhythmias

- *Subcutaneous lidocaine* is used to provide local anesthesia before the placement of a central venous catheter

- *Aerosolized lidocaine* is given before a bronchoscopy is performed

ASSISTING WITH AND PERFORMING RESUSCITATION

Pediatric advanced life support interventions are indicated when the patient has respiratory distress, failure or arrest, and the patient has not successfully responded to initial, basic life support interventions.

RESUSCITATION SITUATIONS

RESPIRATORY ARREST

Pediatric patients are primarily affected with a respiratory arrest prior to a cardiac arrest. These cardiac and respiratory arrests can occur as the result of drowning, choking, poisoning, trauma, sudden infant death syndrome and pneumonia outside of the healthcare environment, and they can also occur as the result of cardiac arrhythmias, respiratory failure, metabolic acidosis and sepsis within or outside of the healthcare facility.

Respiratory arrest occurs primarily from the lack of successful treatment for respiratory distress and respiratory failure. It is characterized by the complete cessation of all breathing, although severe gasping and agonal respirations are also indications of respiratory arrest.

RESPIRATORY DISTRESS

Respiratory distress can occur from a wide variety of cardiopulmonary causes within and outside of the healthcare environment.

The signs and symptoms of respiratory distress include tachycardia, tachypnea, decreased level of consciousness, central cyanosis, apnea, retractions, diaphoresis, grunting, stridor and retractions.

RESPIRATORY FAILURE

Respiratory failure is the presence of inadequate ventilation, inadequate oxygenation or a combination of both.

Some of the underlying causes of respiratory failure are neuromuscular disorders, a number of respiratory diseases and complications, lung disease, a closed head injury and the adverse effect of a medication such as an anesthetic agent. Respiratory failure is immediately treated; there is no need to even check the arterial blood gases until the patient is treated and stabilized.

SELECTING EQUIPMENT

CRASH CARTS

Crash carts are mobile units that are stocked with all the supplies and equipment that is, or may be, necessary for basic and advanced life support. Crash carts must be checked periodically and maintained so that the contents are complete and not expired, and placed in proper areas. The components of the crash cart include:

- *Medications and supplies*

- *Intubation supplies/equipment*

- *Intravenous supplies/equipment*

- *Laboratory supplies/equipment*

- *Procedure-related supplies/equipment*

Medications and Medication Supplies

The medications contained in the crash cart should include Amiodarone, atropine, sodium bicarbonate, calcium chloride, lidocaine, sodium chloride, dextrose 50%, dopamine, epinephrine, vasopressin, alcohol swabs and sterile water. Specific pediatric medications include the following in these preparations:

- *Atropine 0.5 mg/ 5 ml syringe*

- *Sodium Bicarbonate 10 mEq/ 10 ml syringe*

- *Sodium Chloride 0.9% 10 ml flush syringe*

Intubation Supplies and Equipment

The following pediatric intubation supplies and equipment are stocked in the crash cart.

- *Pediatric Stylet (8 Fr)*

- *Neonatal Stylet (6 Fr)*

- *Laryngoscope Blades*

- *Disposable Miller Blades*

- *Disposable Macintosh Blade*

- *Pediatric suction catheters of various sizes*

- *A source of suction*

- *Yankauer suction*

- *2.5 mm Un-cuffed endotracheal tube*

- *3.0mm – 5.5 mm Micro-cuff endotracheal tubes*

- *Nasopharyngeal and perhaps oropharyngeal airways*

- *A flashlight with extra batteries*

- *A syringe of sufficient size to inflate the endotracheal tube cuff*

- *Bite block*

- *Tongue depressors*

- *Supplies to start waveform capnography*

Intravenous Supplies and Equipment

These supplies and equipment include:

- *Umbilical vessel catheter*

- *Disinfectants (swab sticks)*

- *Pediatric IV kits*

- *Pediatric cut down kit*

- *IV tubing*

- *IV solutions*

- *Luer lock syringes of various sizes*
- *Tourniquet tubing*
- *Insyte Auto-guards of various sizes*
- *Arm-boards of various sizes*
- *3-Way stopcock*

Laboratory Supplies and Equipment

Laboratory supplies and equipment such as the following are also stocked in the crash cart.

- *Vacutainers for blood collection*
- *Spinal needles*
- *Bone marrow needles of various sizes*
- *Spinal needles of various sizes*
- *Lumbar puncture kit*
- *Regular needles of various sizes*
- *ABG syringes and sampling kits*

PROCEDURE-RELATED SUPPLIES AND EQUIPMENT

- *ECG machine and electrodes*
- *Sterile gloves of all sizes*
- *Sutures of various sizes and materials*
- *Salem pump*
- *Cricothyroidotomy kit*
- *Sterile drapes*
- *Large bore needle and syringe for tension pneumothorax*

T-PIECE RESUSCITATORS

T-Piece resuscitation devices, which are manufactured by a number of companies, provide the patient with controlled target peak inspiratory pressure (PIP) and positive end expiratory pressure (PEEP) to improve and increase lung volume and improve the patient's functional residual capacity (FRC.)

Scientific controlled trials among newborns compared this device to the self-inflating bag resuscitator, discussed below, and there were no differences in terms of the neonate's morbidity and mortality outcomes; however, many consider the T-piece resuscitators superior because they can deliver pressures closer to the determined target pressure and they have a greater ability to deliver prolonged inflation breaths that are more consistent with the tidal volumes. In summary, T-piece resuscitators can provide free flow oxygen through the mask and a consistent pre-set inspiratory pressure and positive end-expiratory pressure.

Some of the disadvantages of the T-piece, when compared to other methods of resuscitation, include the time necessary for set up and adjusting pressures during resuscitation, in addition to the fact that they may have larger mask leaks and less of an ability to detect changes in lung compliance.

FLOW-INFLATING RESUSCITATION BAGS

Although self-inflating resuscitation bags are an old tradition, they have some advantages over the use of a T-piece resuscitation device and, according to recent research, they are just as effective. Some of the advantages include the fact that an infinite supply of air is available when central supplies and tanks are empty or failed, as can often occur with an internal or external disaster and evacuation or utility failure. It is also portable and, because of this feature, it can be used anywhere inside and outside of the medical facility.

PROTOCOLS

EVIDENCE BASED PRACTICE GUIDELINES

Simply stated, evidence based practice begins with research and then this research is applied to the development of evidence based practice guidelines which are disseminated through a wide variety mechanisms including publications and professional conferences. These evidence based practice guidelines can, and should, be applied to practice after the research and the guidelines are critiqued by the respiratory care professional. Some areas of consideration for integrating evidence based practices into one's role include:

- *Is the evidence-based practice feasible and practical?*

- *Do the potential benefits outweigh the possible risks and costs?*

- *Is it effective and efficient?*

Providing an evidence-based approach to care requires that you can:

- *Access and appraise evidence (research findings)*

- *Understand relationships between research and the strength of evidence*

- *Determine applicability to a patient's condition, context and wishes.*

Some of the databases that healthcare professionals can use regularly to review research and evidence based practice are listed below along with the internet link:

- The Cochrane Library[1]

- The Agency for Healthcare Research and Quality National Guideline Clearing House[2]

- The Joanna Briggs Institute[3]

- Ovid's Evidence Based Medicine Reviews (EBMR)[4]

- Medlars[5]

- Medline Plus (An International nursing index and Index Medicus is also included)[6]

- Pub Med[7]

- The Cumulative Index to Nursing and Allied Health Literature (CINAHL)[8]

- The Directory of Open Access Journals (Free)[9]

- The American Heart Association[10]

- The Neonatal Resuscitation Program (NRP)[11]

[1] http://www.thecochranelibrary.com/view/0/AboutTheCochraneLibrary.html

[2] http://www.guideline.gov/

[3] http://www.joannabriggs.edu.au/

[4] http://www.ovid.com/webapp/wcs/stores/servlet/ProductDisplay?storeId=13051&catalogId=13151&langId=-1&partNumber=Prod-904410

[5] http://www.nlm.nih.gov/bsd/mmshome.html

[6] http://www.nlm.nih.gov/medlineplus/

[7] http://www.ncbi.nlm.nih.gov/pubmed/

[8] http://www.ebscohost.com/cinahl/)

[9] http://www.doaj.org

[10] https://donate.heart.org

[11] http://www2.aap.org/nrp/about.html

PALS

The American Heart Association has developed guidelines, protocols and a certification program for Pediatric Advanced Life Support (PALS.) The PALS algorithms and procedures are considered the gold standard of pediatric resuscitation. According to PALS, the signs and symptoms of severe or complete airway obstruction include:

- *Cyanosis*

- *Weak or ineffective cough*

- *High-pitched/no sound at inspiration*

- *Distressed/difficult breathing*

- *Inability to cry and/or speak*

- *The universal choking sign (fingers around the neck)*

THE NEONATAL RESUSCITATION PROGRAM (NRP)

The Neonatal Resuscitation Program (NRP) is joint program of the American Academy of Pediatrics and the American Heart Association (AHA.) This program and their pediatric resuscitation program are based on current evidence based research and guidelines and protocols.

GENERAL CARE

In addition to providing critical care services to pediatric patients, respiratory therapists also provide acute and sub-acute care in healthcare facilities and in the community.

This section will discuss many of these pediatric services and the role of the respiratory therapist in the assessment, planning, implementation and evaluation of this care.

ASSESSING PATIENT STATUS AND CHANGES IN STATUS

SPECIFIC AIRWAY CHALLENGES

Respiratory therapists face specific airway challenges every day. Some of the most commonly occurring challenges are caring for and treating patients with:

- *Acute upper airway obstruction*
- *Congenital anomalies*

ACUTE UPPER AIRWAY OBSTRUCTION

For the purpose of this discussion, an upper airway obstruction is one that occurs from the nose and mouth to the main carina. Acute disorders, including upper airway obstructions, are different from chronic disorders in that acute disorders have a rapid onset rather than a gradual one. Acute upper airway obstructions can occur as the result of:

- *Foreign body aspiration*

- *Penetrating and blunt laryngotracheal trauma*

- *Tonsillar hypertrophy*

- *Peritonsillar abscess*

- *Laryngotracheobronchitis (Croup)*

- *Paralysis of the vocal cord*

- *Tracheitis*

- *Epiglottitis*

- *Pertussis*

- *Retropharyngeal abscess*

Foreign Body Aspiration

The pediatric population is at risk for foreign body placements into orifices of the body such as the nose, mouth, ear and eyes. Acute upper airway obstruction can occur when a foreign body like food, a small toy or another object is placed in the mouth or nose.

Some of the signs and symptoms of a respiratory tract obstruction are apnea, coughing, agitation, cyanosis, unconsciousness, panic, air hunger and unusual respiratory noises such as crowing, whistling and wheezing.

Emergency measures, such as the Heimlich maneuver, are done with a complete airway obstruction. Other treatments include oxygen administration, foreign body removal, an endotracheal or nasotracheal tube and mechanical ventilation, as indicated.

Penetrating and Blunt Laryngotracheal Trauma

Penetrating and blunt laryngotracheal trauma, as well as multiple trauma, can occur with a number of environmental injuries including a bomb blast or an automobile accident.

The signs and symptoms of a penetrating laryngotracheal trauma can include a visual presence of an open airway; the same visual presence is not present with a blunt trauma - however, bruising and other signs of evident facial, thoracic and total body trauma may be obvious until a diagnosis of laryngotracheal trauma is made. Varying degrees of respiratory compromise will be present depending on the severity of this and other traumas that the patient has suffered. Patients with trauma are assessed by the emergency department staff and/or the emergency first responders in the field. This assessment consists of a physical examination and the history of the trauma.

After the ABC's and any life threatening injuries and conditions are assessed for and treated, further treatments are indicated.

Tonsillar Hypertrophy

Tonsillar hypertrophy, or tonsillar enlargement, occurs as a result of an infection such as a streptococcal infection. It is also referred to as tonsillitis.

The signs and symptoms are a sore throat, fever, exudative pharyngitis and cervical adenopathy. A viral infection, rather than a bacterial infection, is signaled when a cough and/or nasal congestion is present. Rapid streptococcal antigen testing or a throat culture is done to make the definitive diagnosis.

This acute infection is treated with antibiotics when it is bacterial; interventions to reduce the fever and providing the child with respiratory and bodily comfort and support also help.

Peritonsillar Abscess

Peritonsillar abscesses are acute infections that are typically found unilaterally – that is, affecting one tonsil.

The signs of a peritonsillar abscess are a protrusion and swelling of one tonsil into the oropharynx. It is also accompanied with a deviation of the uvula toward the unaffected tonsil, trismus, torticollis, a hoarse voice and a sore throat. It is diagnosed with physical inspection, a culture and an x-ray when indicated.

The treatment is similar to that of tonsillitis and in the long term, a tonsillectomy is considered.

Acute Laryngotracheobronchitis (Croup)

Croup is primarily caused by the type 1 para-influenza viruses; however, this infection can also be caused by the respiratory syncytial virus (RSV), influenza viruses A and B, adenovirus, Mycoplasma pneumonia, measles, enterovirus and the rhinovirus.

Children from 6 months of age up to three years old are at greatest risk for croup but older children can also be at risk when the influenza virus is the offending microorganism.

The signs and symptoms of croup occur as the result of the inflammation of the trachea, larynx, bronchi, bronchioles and lung parenchyma. Airway obstruction and an increased work of breathing occurs as the result of this swelling, particularly in the subglottic area.

These signs and symptoms, which are typically more pronounced during the nighttime hours, include hypercapnia, atelectasis when the bronchioles become obstructed, a spasmodic, barking cough, hoarseness, possible fever, inspiratory stridor, respiratory distress, tachypnea and retractions; cyanosis and shallow, ineffective respiration can occur in severe cases when the patient tires as the result of increased work of breathing.

The diagnosis is made based on the signs and symptoms after other mimicking disorders like epiglottitis, tracheitis and the presence of a foreign body in the airway are ruled out. A chest x-ray will reveal subepiglottic narrowing, also referred to as the steeple sign.

The severity of croup is now scored using the Croup Scoring System, which has measurements, or indicators, of severity such as inspiratory stridor, air entry, cyanosis, retractions and level of consciousness sub-scores ranging from 0 to 5.

Typical treatments include hydration, antipyretics when indicated, humidified cool air, corticosteroids, and at times, humidified oxygen and racemic epinephrine. When the Paco2 is more than 45 mm Hg, endotracheal intubation is indicated.

Paralysis of the Vocal Cord

Paralysis of the vocal cords, which can lead to problems with breathing, swallowing and speaking, typically occurs as the result of a lesion along the neural path of the larynx, trauma or an unknown cause. Women are at more risk than males and it occurs in the left vocal cord more often than the right.

This paralysis can be unilateral or bilateral. Unilateral paralysis typically affects only the voice; bilateral paralysis can completely affect and obstruct the airway and lead to death if not treated.

The signs and symptoms include a hoarse, breathy voice, other alteration of phonation, stridor, dyspnea and difficulty swallowing, which places the patient at risk for aspiration. It is diagnosed with laryngoscopy, the signs and symptoms and MRI imaging.

Patients affected with bilateral paralysis often need intubation until they are further treated and stabilized. Patients with unilateral vocal cord paralysis are most often treated with voice augmentation techniques such as the injection of autologous fat or collagen into the affected cord to bring the cords closer together. Alternatively, some patients may also have voice improvement treatments with re-innervation and medialization procedures.

Unlike those with unilateral paralysis who are treated with surgical procedures to move the cords closer to each other, those with bilateral paralysis are treated with surgical procedures to maintain a patent airway. A permanent or temporary tracheotomy may be needed; an arytenoidectomy with lateralization can be done to open the glottis and improve the patency of the airway but the voice may be adversely affected with this procedure. A posterior laser cordectomy is also done.

Tracheitis

Tracheitis is a true medical emergency that can lead to severe and complete airway obstruction and death. This infection is typically caused by a bacteria.

The signs and symptoms of bacterial tracheitis are a history of a previous upper respiratory infection, fever, elevated white blood cell count that has a high percentage of immature white cells (bands) and a generalized appearance of acute illness and fatigue. The chest and neck x-rays may show irregular mucosal surfaces and the narrowing of the subglottic airway.

The treatment includes an artificial airway and antibiotics to treat the infection; racemic epinephrine is not effective. Because this infection resolves slowly and more slowly than epiglottitis, the airway is typically left in place for at least one week.

Epiglottitis

Similar to tracheitis, epiglottitis is also a life threatening infection. This bacterial infection causes inflammation and swelling of the supraglottic tissues, marked and often very sudden swelling of the epiglottis and surrounding areas, and complete airway obstruction and death if left untreated.

The most common offending microorganism is Haemophilus influenzae type B; however, the incidence of this childhood infection has significant decreased since the advent of the immunization against is Haemophilus influenzae type B.

The onset of symptoms can be very rapid; within only a couple of hours. The signs and symptoms include a high fever, cough, stridor, retracting, drooling, anxiety, a muffled voice and a preference for an upright sitting position with the chin forward. A lateral x-ray will reveal epiglottic folds, which is referred to as the thumb sign, a distended hypopharynx and thickening of the inflamed epiglottis.

The treatment includes the immediate placement of an artificial airway; the size of the endotracheal tube is usually about one size smaller than the expected size to accommodate for the swelling in the upper airway. Once placed, this artificial airway is left in place at least 12-48 hours until the risk of swelling is gone and an air lead of 20 cm H2O occurs around the endotracheal tube.

Short term antibiotics to treat the infection, such as chloramphenicol or ceftriaxone, are given and, if mechanical ventilation is necessary, the child is typically sedated.

Pertussis (Whooping Cough)

Bordetella pertussis is transmitted with respiratory droplets and with direct contact. Whooping cough is transmissible from 7 days after initial exposure through 3 weeks after the coughing has begun. The incubation period ranges from 3 to 12 days after exposure. Pertussis mortality rates are greatest among infants less than 6 months of age. The duration of this infection is about 7 or 8 weeks but the cough can persist for months; it can be prevented with routine immunization. The signs and symptoms vary according to the phase, or stage, of this infectious disease, as follows:

I.   *Catarrhal Stage*

Increased lacrimation, a mild cough, rhinorrhea, conjunctivitis, and a low grade fever

II. *Paroxysmal Stage*

Vomiting, malaise, fatigue, severe whooping coughing leading to cyanosis and exhaustion. The whoop is constant, rapid, consecutive coughs followed by a hurried, deep inspiration.

III. *Convalescent Stage*

Coughing subsides

Pertussis is diagnosed with special nasopharyngeal cultures. Bed rest, a quiet environment, increased fluid intake, the administration of erythromycin estolate, azithromycin, or clarithromycin and respiratory suctioning and supplemental oxygen, as indicated.

Retropharyngeal Abscess

Retropharyngeal abscesses, most common among young children from 1 to 8 years of age, as well as those with tuberculosis and/or HIV, is an infection that develops behind the pharynx in the adjacent retropharyngeal lymph nodes. These abscesses typically occur as the result of a nearby infection affecting the nose, adenoids, sinuses or pharynx. The most common offending organisms include aerobic streptococcus/staphylococcus, anaerobic bacteria and fusobacterium bacteria.

The most serious complications of these abscesses are septic shock, airway obstruction, carotid rupture, aspiration pneumonia, asphyxia, and Lemierre syndrome, which is mediastinitis and thrombophlebitis affecting the internal jugular veins.

The signs and symptoms are a fever, sore throat, odynophagia, dysphagia, cervical lymph node enlargement, adenopathy, nuchal rigidity, stridor, dyspnea, snoring-like noisy breathing and torticollis. A definitive diagnosis is made with a lateral neck x-ray or CT. The posterior pharyngeal wall may bulge to one side. Lateral x-rays of the neck with hyperextension and upon inspiration may reveal air in the pre-vertebral soft tissues, erosion of the nearby vertebral body and widening of the pre-vertebral soft tissues. CT can help differentiate between an abscess and cellulitis, as well as determine the extent and severity of the abscess.

The treatments include surgical drainage and antibiotics like ceftriaxone, a broad-spectrum cephalosporin or clindamycin. Patients who have had surgical drainage are intubated and maintained for about 48 hours after surgery.

Congenital Anomalies

Some congenital anomalies affect the infant's respiratory status upon birth. The treatments for these congenital disorders, in addition to surgical corrections when possible, are as follows:

- *Choanal Atresia:* Oral airway

- *Pierre Robin Syndrome*: Oral or nasal airway and a prone position

- *Periglottic Lesions*: Surgical repairs as indicated for each of these disorders

- *Subglottic Stenosis*: Surgical repair

- *Laryngomalacia*: Self-limiting; disappears within one year or two after birth

- *Tracheal Stenosis*: Surgical correction, however, symptoms may remain postoperatively

Some alternatives for the management of the airway for these challenges are:

- *Anterior commissure intubation*

- *Emergency tracheotomy*

- *Flexible fiber optic intubation*

For more information, see the table on the next page.

Congenital Anomaly	Description	Signs and Symptoms
Choanal Atresia	The absence or stenosis of the nasal passages	Respiratory distress lessened with crying; inability to suction neonate with oropharynx.
Pierre Robin Syndrome	The tongue occludes the airway because the child has a very small oropharynx and a small mandible	Respiratory distress even with crying
Periglottic Lesions	These congenital lesions an include cysts, laryngeal webs, vocal cord paralysis and subglottic hemangiomas.	Respiratory distress and other abnormal signs and symptoms depending on the specific lesion and its severity.
Subglottic Stenosis	Narrowing of the subglottic area	Respiratory distress
Laryngoma-lacia	The arytenoids process and the epiglottis is overly large and floppy	High pitched stridor
Tracheal Stenosis	Narrowing of the trachea that occurs as the result of the aorta wrapping around the trachea and esophagus	Biphasic wheezing, poor feeding, mucus pooling and rhonchi. Characteristic vascular rings of cartilage are present.

CHEST IMAGING

Diagnostic chest imaging is highly useful to respiratory therapists and other healthcare providers in terms of diagnosis and monitoring the patient after diagnosis, when treatments and interventions have begun.

TYPES OF IMAGING STUDIES

- *X-rays*
- *Fluoroscopy*
- *Computed tomography*
- *CT angiography*

- *Magnetic resonance (MRI)*
- *Nuclear scanning*
- *Ultrasonography*

X-rays

X-rays used to image the chest and assess pulmonary status include a simple x-ray, fluoroscopy, CT angiography and high resolution and spiral or helical CT. The most common imaging study for the majority of pulmonary patients is a simple chest x-ray.

Plain chest x-rays and fluoroscopy image the lungs and surrounding structures. Plain chest x-rays images, most often the initial imaging study, allow the identification and diagnosis of a number of abnormalities including those related to the hilum, the mediastinum, the pleura, the chest wall, the diaphragm, the lung parenchyma and the heart.

Standard chest x-rays can be done with a lateral, anterior posterior, an oblique view, and with an end expiratory view. The oblique view is useful to assess the pulmonary nodules and to rule out abnormalities that occur due to superimposed structural images. The lateral view, although not as effective as a CT, provides data relating to pleural effusion; an end expiratory x-ray can provide information about small pneumothoraxes. Lastly, a screening chest x-ray is done when a patient has a positive tuberculin skin test without any symptoms.

Fluoroscopy

Chest fluoroscopy, unlike the simple chest x-ray, uses a continuous beam to image movements of the thoracic region. This continuous x-ray beam is used for the identification of a paralyzed hemidiaphragm. For example, a hemidiaphragm that is paralyzed will move paradoxically and cranially, while a normal and unimpaired hemidiaphragm will be seen as moving caudally, or towards the fluoroscopy.

Computed Tomography (CT)

Similar to a simple chest x-ray, computed tomography images thoracic abnormalities and structures but with a more clear and refined image within multiple 10 mm thick cross-sectional images. It is relatively inexpensive and highly available in the healthcare environment, however, its disadvantages include motion artifacts, and compromised detail and clarity with some tissue.

High-resolution computed tomography, also referred to as HRCT, gives a 1 mm thick cross sectional image, typically during full inspiration, in order to facilitate the best possible images of the airways, the lung's vasculature and the lung parenchyma. It is highly useful for detecting and evaluating obliterative bronchiectasis and interstitial lung disorders such as sarcoidosis, alveolitis and lymphangitic carcinomatosis, masses, infiltrates and fibrosis. HRCT images can also distinguish between dependent atelectasis and other atelectasis.

Spiral or helical computed tomography, done while the patient hold their breath for about 10 seconds, gives us multiple images of the entire chest while the patient is moved gradually and continuously through the CT scanning device. Some of the advantages of spiral or helical computed tomography, when compared to the traditional and conventional CT, include less exposure to radiation, speed, its ability to produce three-dimensional images and to create a virtual bronchoscopy with the help of specialized software. The most recent multi-detector CT machines allow for even more rapid scanning and imaging of thinner slices at higher resolution.

CT Angiography

CT angiography uses an intravenous radiopaque dye and is useful examine pulmonary arteries and diagnose pulmonary embolus. Its benefits include being less invasive and more rapid than conventional angiography, highly accurate in detecting pulmonary emboli.

MRI

A magnetic resonance imaging (MRI) study is a highly detailed evaluation of the chest, which includes the heart, major vessels, mediastinum, lungs, and chest wall. It is more expensive than other diagnostic imaging procedures. Contraindications to MRI include morbidly obese patients and patients with a device, such as cardiac pacemaker or intracranial aneurysm clips, dependent upon metallurgical composition.

Although MRI is relatively limited in terms of pulmonary imaging, it is preferred for the detection of tumors, pulmonary hypertension and cysts, and among patients with an intolerance to contrast dye when a pulmonary embolus is suspected.

The disadvantages of MRI include the time needed for this imaging test, the presence of cardiac and respiratory movements and its contraindications for some patients. Among the advantages of MRI are the absence of bone artifacts, the lack of exposure to radiation and its ability to provide superior images of the vascular structures.

Ultrasonography

Ultrasonography is often used to facilitate procedures such as thoracentesis and central venous catheter insertion, but it is also used for the diagnosis of pulmonary disorders such as a pleural effusion.

Nuclear Scanning

Nuclear scanning techniques used to image the chest include:

- *Ventilation/Perfusion (V/Q) scanning,*

- *Positron emission tomography (PET)*

- *A perfusion (Q) scan*

Ventilation/perfusion, or V/Q, scanning entails intravenous radionuclide to assess perfusion and the inhalation of a radionuclide to assess ventilation. Specifically, areas of perfusion without ventilation and areas of ventilation without perfusion can be visualized with six to eight lung views.

This test is indicated when poor perfusion is suspected, as can be the case with bronchial obstructions secondary to the aspiration of a foreign body, another bronchial obstruction, and an alveolar disorder such as consolidation, atelectasis or emphysema.

A perfusion (Q) scan is done after the intravenous administration of radioactive technetium. This radioactive scan is indicated when an under-perfusion of the pulmonary circulation is suspected. Such under-perfusion can occur as the result of a tumor, a pulmonary embolism and/or pulmonary hypertension.

Normal ventilation and perfusion has a 1:1 ratio of blood and air in the alveoli; a pulmonary embolism leads to a V/Q ratio of >2: 1 which indicates that the ventilation is normal and the perfusion is absent or reduced; airway obstructions, such as that which can occur as the result of atelectasis, have a V/Q ratio of 1 or <1: 2 or >2 because the perfusion is normal and the ventilation is absent or reduced.

Positron emission tomography or PET uses fluorodeoxyglucose to assess and measure the metabolic activity in tissues. It is used to determine the metabolism of the heart and the brain, to determine pulmonary perfusion and ventilation, to determine the size and extent of a myocardial infarction and to metabolically stage tumors without the need for more invasive staging methods that involve, for example, a needle biopsy and a mediastinoscopy.

Position emission tomography (PET) creates images of metabolic tissues by injecting small amounts of a radioactive tracer into the patient. The PET detects metabolic cellular changes and can help identify rapidly growing cells like those associated with lung cancer.

RESPIRATORY PHYSIOLOGY AND MECHANICS

INDICES

Some of the indices of respiratory physiology and mechanics include:

- *Levels of oxygenation*
- *The work of breathing*
- *The results of sleep studies*

Levels of Oxygenation

Arterial blood gases are also used to assess and monitor the patient's improvements or deteriorations in terms of their levels of oxygenation.

The Work of Breathing

The work of breathing is defined as the amount of energy that a person must expend in order to inhale; it is facilitated or impeded by the thoracic cavity, the visceral pleura, the lungs and the parietal pleura. Little effort is needed for exhalation. Patients adversely affected with stiff lungs and/or high airway resistance need more energy to inhale when compared to normal patients. Respirations are regulated by the medulla oblongata, the chemoreceptors, the levels of carbon dioxide, and the pH of the patient.

Normal respiratory ranges and movements normally vary when the patient is an infant or a young child. The newborn typically has silent abdominal signs of respirations that are gentle, shallow and quiet and irregular in terms of rate, rhythm and depth; they also vary from 30 to 60 BPM, usually according to the infant's level of activity; and they occur as the result of the muscles of the diaphragm and the abdomen. As with other measures and assessments, the work of breathing is an indication of the patient's respiratory functioning. Increases indicate deteriorating respiratory functioning and decreases indicate improvement.

The Results of Sleep Studies

Apnea Monitoring

Apnea monitoring is most often used among infants and for other sleep studies that diagnose and monitor patients with sleep apnea. Apnea monitors typically have three alarms. These alarms sound when tachycardia, bradycardia and apnea occur. Neonate apnea monitors are usually set to alarm for a cardiac rate of less than 80 per minute and more than 210 per minute as well as 15 seconds of apnea. These settings are changed as the neonate grows older.

Overnight Pulse Oximetry

Overnight pulse oximetry is measured with a pulse oximetry monitor during the night to measure and record the patient's Spo2, or oxygen saturation, of capillary blood. Pulse oximetry determines the oxygen saturation of this capillary blood by emitting light through diodes that are placed over the patient's fingertip. These levels are accurate within 5% of directly measured Sao2 levels.

This oximetry is typically done most often among patients who are being diagnosed for possible sleep apnea.

POLYSOMNOGRAPHY

Polysomnography, a sleep study, is a highly beneficial way to diagnose and monitor patients who are possibly adversely affected with a sleep or wakefulness disorder like narcolepsy, sleep apnea, nocturnal seizures and/or periodic limb movements. Polysomnography monitors and measures cardiac rate, O2 saturation, brain activity with an electroencephalogram, or EEG, eye movements, respirations, muscle tone and activity while the patient is asleep. These sleep studies are most often conducted in a community-based sleep laboratory; however, at times, they can be done in the patient's home.

There are two types of sleep apnea, namely central and obstructive sleep apnea. Central sleep apnea is characterized by periods of apnea or shallow breathing lasting 10 or more seconds during sleep. This sleep disorder results from impaired and diminished respiratory effort. Obstructive sleep apnea, on the other hand, is characterized by a complete or partial closure of the upper respiratory tract, and sleep apnea of more than ten seconds. This most commonly occurring type of sleep apnea is typically accompanied by snoring.

In addition to polysomnography, a sleep latency test can be performed for patients with possible narcolepsy. A sleep latency test evaluates the patient's ability to initiate sleep during day time nap opportunities. These naps are done two hours apart and, typically, five nap opportunities are used for this test. The patient's onset and stage of sleep are monitored and measured using polysomnography.

NEUROLOGIC STATUS

RESPIRATORY FUNCTION

Neuromuscular control of respiration is well established. This control is the result of the functioning of the CNS and the peripheral nervous system (PNS.) The role of the CNS, which is comprised of the brain and the spinal cord, includes voluntary respirations as innervated by the brain's cerebral cortex and the corticospinal region; involuntary ventilation is innervated by the brain's brainstem and the reticulospinal region. Any dysfunction between the brain and the respiratory muscles impairs the respiratory system and can lead to respiratory failure. The PNS receives signals from the CNS; these PNS neurons then transmit signals to the muscles of respiration.

Any PNS impairment can lead to impaired respiratory functioning because the main inspiratory muscle, the diaphragm, the expiratory muscles such as the internal intercostals and the accessory abdominal muscles and/or the accessory muscles of respiration including the scalene, trapezii, latissimus dorsi, the sternocleidomastoid and/or the pectoralis group may be impaired.

Some of the neuromuscular diseases and disorders that affect the respiratory system and its functioning include:

- *All cranial disorders including brain trauma and swelling*

- *Spinal cord injuries*

- *Poliomyelitis*

- *Spinal muscular atrophy (SMA)*

- *Guillain-Barre syndrome*

- *Infantile botulism*

- *Myasthenia gravis*

- *Duchenne and Becker MD*

- *Myotonic dystrophies*

- *Glycogen storage diseases*

- *Electrolyte disorders*

OTHER DISORDERS

Apnea of Prematurity

The defining criteria of apnea of prematurity is respiratory pauses of more than 20 seconds or an airflow interruption and respiratory pauses more than 20 seconds with bradycardia of less than 80 BPM, cyanosis, or an O2 saturation of less than 85% in neonates less than 37 weeks of gestation without any underlying disorder that could cause the apnea. Approximately 25% of premature infants have apnea of prematurity. It rarely occurs during the first day of life; it begins two or three days after birth. When apnea develops after the 14th day of life it signals another serious disorder like sepsis, rather than apnea of prematurity.

Apnea of prematurity can be classified as obstructive, central and the most common type which is a mixed pattern of apnea of prematurity. The risk factor associated with apnea of prematurity is prematurity and the risk increases with decreasing gestational age.

Central apnea is associated with medullary respiratory control center immaturity and lack of development; obstructive apnea is associated with an obstructed airflow secondary to reflex laryngospasm, nasal occlusion and neck flexion that compresses the hypopharyngeal soft tissues.

Apnea is characterized by cyanosis, hypoxemia and bradycardia, particularly when the period of the apnea is prolonged. The diagnosis is confirmed with cardiac and respiratory monitoring using an impedance cardiorespiratory monitor, for example, that revels apnea as defined above. A differential diagnosis is also made when other possible causes like gastroesophageal reflux disease, hypoglycemia, intracranial hemorrhage and sepsis have been ruled out.

The treatment of central apnea includes the use of tactile stimulation and respiratory stimulants, such as caffeine, and the treatment of obstructive apnea includes the positioning of the neonate's head to relieve the obstruction. The neonate should be positioned on their back with the head midline and the neck slightly extended or in a neutral position to correct upper airway obstruction.

The initial dose of caffeine is 10 mg/kg; the maintenance dose is 2.5 mg/kg po every 24 hours. Alternatively, caffeine citrate with a loading dose 20 mg/kg and a maintenance dose of 5 to 10 mg/kg every 24 hours can be used but caffeine is the drug of choice because it is safer, requires less monitoring and more easily administered than caffeine citrate. Continuous positive airway pressure with a pressure of 5 to 8 cm H2O pressure and ventilator support may be indicated when the apnea does not resolve with other treatments.

Level of Consciousness

Levels of consciousness can change as the result of several causes, some of which are structural and some of which are classified as metabolic. Examples of biological causes of decreased levels of consciousness include infections, cancer including brain tumors, intracerebral hemorrhage, other vascular insults like a cerebrovascular accident, and trauma like a closed head injury. Some metabolic causes of decreased levels of consciousness include seizures, hypoxic encephalopathy, as caused by heart failure and hypertension, systemic metabolic problems like hypoglycemia and ketoacidosis, toxins, and changes in body temperature with extremes of hyperthermia and hypothermia.

The six levels of consciousness are alert, confused, lethargic, obtunded, stuporous and comatose. Alert patients follow commands and answer questions appropriately with minimal stimulation; confused patients are not oriented to their environment, they may lack good judgment and need cues in order to respond to commands; lethargic patients are drowsy but can be rousted with verbal or tactile stimulation; obtunded patients respond slowly and only with repeated stimulation; stuporous patients minimally respond to vigorous stimulation and they may only verbally respond with a moan; lastly, comatose patients are completely unresponsive to external stimuli.

A persistent vegetative state, locked-in syndrome and brain death are three states that are closely associated with altered levels of consciousness. A persistent vegetative state leaves the patient with no cognitive functioning but only basic functions such as a sleep – wake cycle and eye opening. Locked-in syndrome is characterized by retained cognitive functioning but absent motor functioning. In this state, the patient is able to communicate with eye movements and they are typically aware of their surroundings. Brain death is defined as the state where there is a known irreversible cause of the coma, complete unresponsiveness to eternal stimuli, a complete loss of all brainstem reflexes and the absence of respiratory function with the presence of hypercapnia.

The Glasgow Coma Scales for adults and children are standardized assessment tools for altered levels of consciousness. These scales assess motor responses, verbal responses and eye opening. The Rancho Los Amigos scale is used to determine a patient's cognitive level of functioning. This scale ranges from I to VIII, with I as the total lack of all responsiveness to all stimulation and VIII as alert, oriented, appropriate and purposeful.

The Children's Coma Scale is used for infants and toddlers who are developmentally unable to follow commands. This scale measures ocular, verbal and motor responses with a higher numerical score higher levels:

Ocular Responses

4- Active pursuit of the stimulus

3- Reactive pupils, intact extra-ocular movements

2- Fixed pupils, impaired extra-ocular movements

1- Fixed pupils, paralyzed extra-ocular movements

Verbal Responses

3- Infant cries

2- Spontaneous respirations

1- Apnea

Motor Responses

4- Extension and flexion

3- Reacts and withdraws with painful stimuli

2- Hypertonic

1- Flaccid

Treatment includes the correction of the underlying cause, when possible. For example, hypoglycemia can be treated and reversed. When correction of an underlying disorder is not possible, supportive care is indicated.

CARDIOVASCULAR STATUS

HEMODYNAMICS

Hemodynamic monitoring (with and without special indwelling monitoring catheters) provides data and information in respect to a patient's blood pressure, pulmonary artery pressure, pulmonary artery wedge pressure, central venous pressure, cardiac output, intra-arterial pressure and mixed venous oxygen saturation.

Hemodynamic monitoring systems include a pressure transducer, a monitor, pressure tubing a pressure bag and a flush device.

Arterial lines are usually placed in the radial artery and less often in the femoral/brachial arteries. These provide constant data relating to the patient's blood pressure, and also provide access for the drawing of arterial blood samples.

Pulmonary artery catheters, although used less today than in the past, are inserted through the right side of the heart to the pulmonary artery to measure and monitor central venous, or mixed, O2 saturation, cardiac output and preload. These catheters are placed into a large vein such as the femoral, subclavian, brachial or internal jugular veins. Similar to an arterial line, pulmonary artery catheters also provide not only hemodynamic monitoring and assessments, but also lumens that can accommodate venous blood samples and the infusion of intravenous fluids.

Pulmonary artery catheters are indicated for a number of disorders including complicated heart failure, complicated myocardial infarction, ventricular septal rupture, complicated pulmonary emboli, pulmonary hypertension, and hemodynamic instability when volume status must be assessed/monitored, as well as for patients who have had cardiac surgery and/or are critically ill. The components of a pulmonary artery catheter are:

- *The distal lumen,* which measures the pulmonary artery systolic, the pulmonary artery diastolic, and the pulmonary wedge pressure. The distal lumen is NOT used for the administration of intravenous fluids.

- *The proximal lumen,* which measures the central venous pressure (right atrial pressure) is also used for the administration of intravenous fluids and to collect venous blood samples.

- *The balloon inflation port,* which is used to measure pulmonary artery wedge pressure when inflated, is deflated and locked when not being used to measure pulmonary artery wedge pressure.

- *The thermistor,* which is used to determine the cardiac output by comparing the difference between the pulmonary artery and the right atrium of the heart.

The normal values for hemodynamic monitoring aspects, with minor differences among various sources, are as below.

- *Pulmonary Artery Systolic Pressure: 15-26 mm Hg*

- *Pulmonary Artery Diastolic Pressure: 5-15 mm Hg*

- *Pulmonary Artery Wedge Pressure: 4-12 mm Hg*

- *Central Venous Pressure: 1-8 mm Hg*

- *Cardiac Output: 4-7 L/min*

- *Mixed Venous Oxygen Saturation: 60%-80%*

- *Right Atrium Pressure: 0-8 mm Hg*

- *Right Ventricle Peak Systolic: 15-30 mm Hg*

- *Right Ventricle End Diastolic: 0-8 mm Hg*

- *Pulmonary Artery Mean: 9-16 mm Hg*

- *Pulmonary Artery Peak Systolic: 15-30 mm Hg*

- *Pulmonary Artery End Diastolic: 4-14 mm Hg*

- *Pulmonary Artery Occlusion Mean: 2-12 mm Hg*

- *Left Atrium Mean: 2-12 mm Hg*

- *Left Atrium A Wave: 4-16 mm Hg*

- *Left Atrium V Wave: 6-12 mm Hg*

- *Left Ventricle Peak Systolic: 90-140 mm Hg*

- *Left Ventricle End Diastolic: 5-12 mm Hg*

- *Brachial Artery Mean: 70-150 mm Hg*

- *Brachial Artery Peak Systolic: 90-140 mm Hg*

- *Brachial Artery End Diastolic:*   *60-90 mm Hg*

Pulmonary Artery Wedge Pressure

Pulmonary artery wedge pressures are monitored when the pulmonary artery catheter is inflated against the inner aspect of the pulmonary artery. This hemodynamic monitoring is used for a number of conditions and disorders such as a myocardial infarction, heart failure, valve disorders, pulmonary embolus, pulmonary hypertension, pulmonary edema, shock, burns, arterial venous malformations, multi system failure and cardiac tamponade.

Central Venous Pressure

Central venous pressure is the average blood pressure in the veins as measured with the pressure in the thoracic vena cava in close proximity to the right atrium of the heart. Central venous pressure is an important hemodynamic measurement that impacts on the filling pressure, the preload in the right ventricle and stroke volume. Changes in the central venous pressure readings are mathematically determined by dividing the change in volume in the thoracic vein by the compliance of this thoracic vein, therefore, the central venous pressure increases when there is a decrease in venous compliance or an increase in the venous blood volume. Some of the factors that impact on venous blood volume and venous compliance include:

- *Respiratory activity*
- *Gravity*
- *Venous dilating medications*
- *Leg and abdominal skeletal muscle contraction*
- *Cardiac output*

Cardiac Output

Cardiac output, defined as the amount of blood that the heart ejects per minute, normally ranges from 4 to 8 L per minute. Some of the mathematical techniques that calculate the cardiac output include the Fick technique, the indicator dilution technique and the thermo-dilution technique.

The Fick Technique

The Fick technique is based on the premise that cardiac output is proportionate to oxygen consumption divided by the arteriovenous oxygen difference, and is calculated by:

$$CO = \frac{Ambient\ O_2\ -\ Expired\ O_2\ (mL/min)}{(1.36)\ (Hb\ g/dL)\ \times\ (SaO_2\ -\ SvO_2)}$$

The Indicator Dilution Technique

The indicator dilution technique is calculated by:

$$CO = \frac{Injectate\ mass\ (mg)}{\int_\infty C(t)\ dt}$$

The Thermodilution Technique

The thermodilution technique employs the equation below. TB – TI is the difference between the body and the injectate temperature that typically consists of saline or dextrose; and the denominator of this equation is sum of temperature changes for each time interval.

The thermodilution technique and the indicator dilution technique are based on the premise that the injected saline or dextrose will disappear or appear proportionate to the carbon dioxide.

THE CARDIAC INDEX

The cardiac index reflects CO in relationship to the patient's bodily surface area, or BSA. The BSA is calculated using the DuBois method:

$$BSA\ in\ m^2\ =\ (wt\ in\ kg)^{0.425}\ \times\ (ht\ in\ cm)^{0.725}\ \times\ 0.007184$$

This index is expressed in terms of L/min/m2. The normal cardiac index ranges from 3.0 to 4.5 L/min/ m2.

PRELOAD AND AFTERLOAD

Preload, afterload, the amount of adequate myocardium, substrate availability, cardiac rate and cardiac rhythm, in concert, impact on the velocity and force of cardiac contractility, myocardial oxygen needs and ventricular functioning.

Preload, simply stated, is the loading ability of the heart at the end of diastole, or relaxation, just prior to the next systole, or next contraction. Preload is impacted by the condition of the myocardial wall and the ventricular diastolic pressure and it can change or be modified as the result of myocardial compliance, hypertrophy and left ventricular dilation. On most occasions, the left ventricular end diastolic pressure is an accurate measurement of preload, especially when the left ventricular end diastolic pressure is high and elevated.

The Frank-Starling Law describes the relationship between preload and cardiac performance. With other factors remaining constant, the greater the blood volume in the heart's ventricle during the relaxed phase (diastole) the greater the amount of blood that will be moved during systole, or the contraction phase. This is sometimes also referred to as the Maestrini law. In essence, systolic stroke volume is proportionate to the preload.

Afterload, on the other hand, depends on wall thickness, the volume and the chamber pressure at the start of systole when the aortic valve opens and these forces resist myocardial fiber contraction at the start of systole. Systemic systolic BP when the aortic valve opens represents peak systolic wall stress and an approximation of afterload.

Preload Alterations with Elevated Right Heart Central Venous Pressure and Elevated Left Heart Pulmonary Artery Wedge Pressure

- *Peripheral edema*
- *Hepatomegaly*
- *Lung sound crackles*
- *Jugular vein distension*
- *Taut skin*

Preload Alterations with Decreased Right Heart Central Venous Pressure and Decreased Left Heart Pulmonary Artery Wedge Pressure

- *Dry mucous membranes*
- *Poor skin turgor*

Afterload Alterations with Elevated Right Heart Pulmonary Vascular Resistance and Elevated Left Heart Systemic Vascular Resistance

- *Weakened peripheral pulses*
- *Coolness of extremities*

Afterload Alterations Decreased Right Heart Pulmonary Vascular Resistance and Decreased Left Heart Systemic Vascular Resistance

- *Bounding peripheral pulses*
- *Warm extremities*

Pulmonary Hypertension

Pulmonary hypertension is higher-than-normal pressure in pulmonary circulation. Many conditions, such as left heart failure, parenchymal lung disease and sleep apnea, and drugs can lead to pulmonary hypertension. There are five classifications or categories of pulmonary hypertension. Right ventricular overload and failure dyspnea upon exertion, fatigue, syncope and chest discomfort can occur with severe pulmonary hypertension.

Initial testing begins with spirometry, an ECG, chest x-ray and a transthoracic Doppler echocardiography. The final diagnosis is made based on these tests, the signs, symptoms, and elevated pulmonary artery pressure, which can be detected with an ECG and confirmed with right heart catheterization. Clinically, the diagnosis is made when the pulmonary arterial pressure ≥ 25 mm Hg at rest.

Pulmonary hypertension is treated with diuretics and vasodilators, and requires treating any underlying disorder.

RECOGNIZING RESPIRATORY FAILURE MECHANISMS

PRIMARY PULMONARY AND AIRWAY DISEASES

Some of the primary pulmonary and airway disorders and diseases that can lead to respiratory failure include:

- *Atelectasis*
- *Pneumonia*
- *Asthma*
- *Croup*

Atelectasis

Atelectasis is the often reversible collapse of lung tissue that is accompanied with a loss of lung volume. Atelectasis can result from extrinsic and intrinsic airway compression, such as lymphadenopathy and a mucus plug or a foreign body, respectively, poorly placed endotracheal tubes, hypoventilation and cough suppression as can occur with general anesthesia and over sedation, a prolonged supine position and the impairment or collapse of the lung's parenchyma as the result of a pneumothorax or pleural effusion.

Some of the complications associated with atelectasis are pneumonia and compromised respiratory status marked with a ventilation/perfusion [V/Q] mismatch and hypoxia. The body's normal defenses against atelectasis and normal lung functioning are:

- The presence of surfactant to maintain surface tension
- Deep breathing to release surfactant

- Coughing to clear secretions from airway
- Continuous breathing

Signs and symptoms are chest pain, dyspnea and hypoxia symptoms when severe. The diagnosis is usually based on signs, symptoms and a chest x-ray.

The treatment includes coughing and deep breathing using an incentive spirometer. Incentive breathing devices facilitate and motivate, or incentivize, patients to perform hyperinflation therapy. These hyperinflation exercises include coughing and deep breathing to treat and prevent pulmonary infiltrates, pneumonia and atelectasis. These breathing techniques mobilize secretions, which is not only beneficial to patients with pulmonary disorders. Those who will be undergoing surgery should learn coughing and deep breathing exercises prior to surgery, to prevent post-operative pulmonary disorders. Surgical patients are encouraged to splint the incisional site while coughing and deep breathing in order to decrease discomfort.

Incentive spirometers are helpful to patients in terms of these exercises because the patient can visualize their inspiratory capacity with and without the presence of the respiratory therapist. An inspiratory capacity of 80% or more of the preoperative value indicates no need for respiratory treatments unless the chest x-ray shows abnormalities and/or atelectasis exists. Similarly, when the inspiratory capacity is less than 33% of the preoperative value or the vital capacity is less than 10mL/kg, IPPB is indicated.

Pneumonia

Pneumonia is a lower respiratory tract infection that can be caused by a variety of bacteria, including streptococcus pneumonia, viruses, protozoa and fungi. Gram positive bacteria like B. Streptococcus and S. Aureus and gram negative enteric bacilli are the most common causes of pneumonia among neonates. Infants older than 1 month and children up to about 5 years of age are most often infected with a virus like para-influenza, adenovirus and RSVs. Pneumonia can range in seriousness from mild to life-threatening. It is most serious for infants and young children, people older than age 65, and people with underlying health problems or weakened immune systems.

The signs and symptoms of viral and bacterial pneumonia are as follows:

- *Viral pneumonia*: Fever, cough, nasal congestion, coryza, retractions, wheezing, tachypnea, nasal flaring, respiratory distress and rhonchi.

- *Bacterial pneumonia*: The same signs and symptoms as viral pneumonia, however, they tend to be more severe in terms of the fever and respiratory distress.

Other signs and symptoms include muscular aches, fatigue, enlarged lymph nodes, a sore throat and chest pain.

The treatment of pneumonia includes antibiotics that target the offending bacteria, and fluids and oxygen supplementation, as indicated. The treatment of viral pneumonia includes the administration of aerosolized ribavirin (an antiviral drug) and supportive care and monitoring of the arterial blood gases and pulse oximetry to detect any hypercarbia, hypoxemia and respiratory compromise. Extracorporeal oxygenation (ECMO), intubation and mechanical ventilation may be necessary in severe cases.

Asthma

Asthma is the inflammation and the narrowing of the airways. Asthma can be acute or chronic. Severe asthma attacks can be life threatening, therefore, emergency treatment is necessary. Asthma can be acute or chronic and both forms are associated with hyper-secretion of mucus and bronchial hyper-responsiveness.

Some of the risk factors associated with asthma are:

- *Exposures to environmental factors such as allergens, viruses, tobacco smoke, molds, dust mites, cockroaches, carpet irritants and other respiratory irritants.*

- *Pre-pubescent male gender*
- *Post-pubescent female gender*
- *African American and Hispanic ethnicity*
- *Low birth weight infants*
- *Maternal smoking during pregnancy*
- *Atopic dermatitis*

The signs and symptoms of airway obstructions secondary to asthma include acute bronchoconstriction, mucous plugs, dyspnea, chest pain, coughing, wheezing, shortness of breath, airway remodeling, airway hyper-responsiveness, inflammation, chest pain and tightness and airway edema. The components of diagnosis, in addition to a complete medical history and physical examination, include spirometry to assess the pulmonary function and broncho-provocation challenges.

Broncho-provocation challenges for the diagnosis of asthma can use both pharmacologic and non-pharmacological challenges. A pharmacological methacholin challenge is considered positive when there is a 20% or more decrease in the patient's FEV1; a positive exercise challenge and the presence of bronchospasm induced with exercise are confirmed when the FEV1 decreases by 15% or more below the established baseline.

The treatment of asthma aims to prevent chronic asthma, to maintain normal activity levels, maintain pulmonary function, to decrease and prevent exacerbations and to provide the patient with pharmacological agents to manage the asthma that leaves the patient without any adverse effects of side effects.

Severe and emergency cases are treated with B2 agonists, corticosteroids, intubation and mechanical ventilation when indicated by the patient's current condition and respiratory status. Bronchodilators, such as albuterol, levalbuterol and pirbuterol, are used to quickly open swollen airways. Other quick relief medications that are used include ipratropium and oral and IV corticosteroids, such as prednisone.

The National Asthma Education and Prevention Program recommends the following treatments for the management of asthma:

- *Long term control medications such as long acting B2 agonists, anti-inflammatory medications, methylxanthines, leukotriene modifiers, immunomodulators and cromolyn sodium with nedocromil*

- *Quick-relief medications like short acting B2 agonists, corticosteroids and anticholinergic drugs.*

- *The identification and avoidance of triggers*

- *Allergen immunotherapy when indicated*

- *Close monitoring using a peak flow meter, a peak flow diary, a person best reading, a peak flow zone system and an asthma management plan*

OTHER PULMONARY AND AIRWAY DISEASES

Some other pulmonary and airway diseases and disorders include:

- *Neuromuscular disorders and diseases*

- *Respiratory control disorders and diseases*

- *Flail chest*

Neuromuscular Disorders and Diseases

Neuromuscular diseases and disorders that affect the respiratory system and its functioning include:

- *Cranial disorders including brain trauma and swelling*

- *Spinal cord injuries*

- *Poliomyelitis*

- *SMA*

- *Guillain-Barre syndrome*
- *Infantile botulism*
- *Myasthenia gravis*
- *Duchenne and Becker MD*

- *Myotonic dystrophies*
- *Glycogen storage diseases*
- *Electrolyte disorders*

Flail Chest

A flail chest is the separation of a part of the chest wall as the result of several adjacent rib fractures in two areas. This disorder occurs as the result of trauma.

The signs and symptoms include a paradoxical movement of the area with inhalation and expiration. The flail segment moves outward during expiration, and inward during inhalation – the opposite of the normal occurrence during the respiratory cycle. This paradoxical movement impedes normal tidal volume, increases the work of breathing and can cause serious respiratory compromise.

The diagnosis is made with a visual inspection of the chest for paradoxical movement, palpation to detect crepitus and a chest x-ray that confirms rib fractures and some pulmonary contusions.

The treatments depend on the severity of the disorder and the degree of respiratory compromise. Treatments can range from simply supportive care like mild analgesia to supplemental humidified oxygen supplementation to intubation and mechanical ventilation. Pediatric patients with significant flail chest are treated with intubation, positive pressure ventilation and paralysis for 5 to 7 days until the healing begins and the child is stabilized.

RENAL, METABOLIC, ENDOCRINE, AND NUTRITIONAL DISORDERS

Fluid Balance

A patient's fluid balance is defined as the difference between the intake of fluids, which usually includes drinking or intravenous fluids, and fluid outputs, which is primarily from urination, in addition to other non-perceptible losses like sweat and tears.

A positive fluid balance occurs as the result of excessive fluid intake in the form of oral and/or intravenous fluids or a decrease in fluid output, as can occur with renal insufficiency and renal failure. A positive fluid balance can lead to pulmonary edema, peripheral edema and hypertension. A negative fluid balance is usually the result of insufficient hydration and dehydration, excessive urination, severe diarrhea and/or vomiting and as the result of medications such as diuretics or xanthenes like theophylline.

Fluids and the fluid balance is closely monitored by respiratory therapists. Fluid balance is assessed with serum electrolytes, particularly sodium, as well as urine electrolytes and osmolality.

A positive fluid balance, also referred to as extracellular fluid and fluid overload, can lead to pulmonary edema, peripheral edema and hypertension; excessive fluids can result from heart failure, nephrotic syndrome, and cirrhosis. When it results from heart failure, there is decreased effective circulating volume which can lead to decreased organ perfusion.

A negative fluid balance is usually the result of insufficient hydration and dehydration, excessive urination, severe diarrhea and/or vomiting as the result of medications such as diuretics or xanthenes like theophylline.

The signs and symptoms of fluid excesses include weight gain, dependent peripheral edema, pulmonary edema and hypertension. The signs and symptoms of fluid deficits include diminished skin turgor, dry mucous membranes, tachycardia, tachypnea, hypotension (including orthostatic), sunken eyes, thirst, oliguria, confusion, poor capillary refill and weight loss.

Neonatal Fluids and Fluid Values

Dextrose 5% is administered intravenously to neonates weighing less than 1500 g at the rate of 60 to 80 mL/kg/day, but this rate is modified according to the neonate's urinary output and blood glucose levels. These infants will have a urinary catheter to collect and determine their urinary output; frequent electrolyte laboratory tests are done to determine the patient's fluid level, electrolytes and blood glucose. If hyponatremia or "air block" occurs, the Syndrome of Inappropriate Antidiuretic Hormone Secretion, also referred to as SIADH, is rule out or diagnosed with measures of serum and urine osmolality or specific gravity.

The normal urinary output for the infant is 0.5 to 5 mL/kg/hr; the normal blood glucose is from 60 to 80 mg/ dL. When interpreting urine electrolyte and osmolality values, the following should be kept in mind:

During volume depletion, normal functioning kidneys retain sodium, therefore the urine sodium concentration is less than < 15 mEq/L; the fractional excretion of Na is usually < 1% and the urine osmolality is typically more than 450 mOsm/kg. When metabolic alkalosis occurs with volume depletion, the urinary concentration of sodium becomes elevated because large amounts of HCO3 are spilled into the urine. The excretion of sodium occurs and the urine chloride concentration decreases to less than 10 mEq/L. Volume depletion often increases the blood urea nitrogen (BUN) and serum creatinine concentrations with the ratio of BUN: Creatinine often more than 20:1. Additionally, laboratory values like the hematocrit may increase.

Electrolytes

Details about normal levels of electrolytes were previously discussed.

NUTRITION AND FEEDING

NEONATAL NUTRITIONAL NEEDS

Neonates are normally expected to lose up to 10% of their birth weight within a couple of days after delivery but this loss is expected to be regained within 14 days after delivery. Neonates and infants are also expected to gain between 110 to 200 g per week for the first three months of life. The nutritional needs of the neonate include:

- *Calories*: 110 kcal/kg/day for the first 3 months and then 100 kcal/kg/day from 3 to 6 months of age.

- *Fluids*: 140 to 160 mL/kg per day

- *Protein*: 2.25 to 4 g/kg per day

- *Carbohydrates*: From 40 to 50% of the total caloric intake

Non-breast fed infants should be given 400 IU of vitamin D on a daily basis; a minimum of 15% and up to 50% of the caloric intake should be from fats and triglycerides and supplemental water is sometimes indicated. With the exception of fluoride and iron, both breast milk and formulas contain sufficient minerals. Based on this fact, iron and fluoride supplementation are indicated.

BREASTMILK AND BOTTLED FORMULA

Human milk is the best form of nutrition for babies up to at least 6 months of age. It is easily digested and absorbed, and contains bioavailable micronutrients in the proper amount. A pregnant woman must weigh many factors when deciding whether to breastfeed. Some of these factors include employment status, socioeconomic status and life style choices, among others. For example, a woman who has no paid leave time from work after having a baby may elect to bottle feed because they cannot afford to stay home with the baby. The choice to breastfeed is up to the parent(s) after education relating to breastfeeding and formula feeding is provided. Many families decide on this choice prior to delivery; however, this is not always the case. The decision may be made during the postpartum period.

Milk is synthesized, or manufactured, in the epithelial lining of the alveoli and this production is stimulated by prolactin. Prolactin and oxytocin, endocrine hormones produced by the pituitary, regulate milk production.

Component	Breast Milk	Milk Based Formulas
Fluids	About 90% water	About 90% water
Fats	98% to 99% is fat/triglycerides	The amount of fats varies according to the brand.
Carbo-hydrates	The primary carbohydrate is lactose. Other sources of carbohydrates are nitrogen-containing oligosaccharides and glucosamine.	The amount of carbohydrates varies according to the brand. Cow's milk based formula has less carbohydrates than human milk
Protein	Casein and whey are the two proteins found in breast milk. They are referred to as curd and lactalbumin, respectively. Protease and lipase are also contained in breast milk.	Contains more whey than breast milk
Vitamins	Low in vitamin D Rich in vitamins B and C	Fortified with vitamins
Minerals	Meets neonatal requirements of minerals	Meets neonatal requirements of minerals
Trace	Nucleotides, carnitine and	Nucleotides, carnitine

Elements	taurine are present	and taurine are added

The Nutritional Needs of the Ill Neonate

Nutritionally compromised patients need enteral or parenteral nutrition.

Enteral nutrition delivers nourishment and nutrients directly into the gastrointestinal tract with a tube feeding like a nasogastric tube feeding or a gastrostomy tube feeding. Nasogastric tube feedings are the preferred method except when the patient is affected with a swallowing disorder, impaired gag reflex and/or a disorder of the esophageal sphincter which could potentially lead to reflux. When long term enteral feeding is anticipated, a percutaneous endoscopic gastrostomy (PEG) tube is endoscopically introduced into the stomach and through the abdominal wall with the use of a local anesthetic. Enteral nutrition, similar to parenteral nutrition, consists of essential nutrients and many different solutions that vary in terms of their osmolality, calories, and the proportions of fat, carbohydrates and protein, which is the most essential element of all. Solutions are selected as based on the patient's needs. These feedings can be delivered on a continuous basis, intermittently or as a bolus. Complications include bacterial contamination, aspiration, diarrhea, particularly when a high caloric density formula is used, and regurgitation.

Unlike enteral nutrition, parenteral nutrition is delivered intravenously. This method is preferred when the patient needs nutritional support for more than one week. Although this form of nutrition can be delivered through a peripheral vein, it is most often delivered with a central venous catheter and a port. Scrupulous sterile dressing changes must be done in order to prevent infection, which is a commonly occurring complication of parenteral nutrition. Complications associated with parenteral nutrition include tube obstructions, air embolus, infection, and metabolic disturbances like glucose intolerance. An umbilical arterial catheter, if in place for blood sample withdrawal, must be removed before any total parenteral nutrition (TPN) can begin.

ACID-BASE BALANCE

Respiratory therapists closely monitor and assess the patient's acid-base balance because adjustments in terms of ventilator settings and fluids can be made to correct any imbalances of the patient's acid base balance.

The assessment of acid-base balances is done by assessing and interpreting the patient's [H, Paco2 and HCO3 for the presence of any acidosis or alkalosis. The two primary categories of acid-base imbalances are metabolic and respiratory. These two broad categories are further refined as respiratory acidosis, respiratory alkalosis, metabolic acidosis and metabolic alkalosis.

The causes of respiratory acidosis can be related to lung disease, impaired respiratory function, neuromuscular disorders that affect respiratory functioning and other causes as follows:

- *Upper airway obstructions like croup and epiglottitis*
- *Small airway obstructions like asthma and bronchiolitis*
- *Pulmonary edema*
- *Respiratory distress syndrome*
- *Pulmonary hypoplasia*
- *Pulmonary edema*
- *Aspiration of a foreign body or meconium*
- *Pleural effusion*
- *Pneumothorax*
- *Apnea*
- *Thoracic cage disorders like flail chest and osteogenesis imperfecta*
- *Poliomyelitis*
- *Myasthenia gravis*
- *Diaphragmatic paralysis*
- *Brain stem/spinal cord injuries*
- *Guillain-Barre syndrome*
- *Botulism*

Among the causes of respiratory alkalosis are:

- *Hypoxemia related to a number of respiratory causes such as pneumonia, emboli, heart failure, asthma and atelectasis*

- *Mechanical ventilation*

- *Hyperthyroidism*

- *Liver failure*

- *Salicylate poisoning*

- *CNS impairments such as a head injury, a tumor and infection*

The possible causes of metabolic acidosis include:

- *Diabetic ketoacidosis*

- *Renal failure*

- *The ingestion of poisons and toxins including chloride compounds*

- *Hyper alimentation*

- *Diarrhea*

- *Lactic acidosis secondary to tissue hypoxia*

The causes of metabolic alkalosis include:

- *Infants with cystic fibrosis fed with breast milk or regular formula*

- *Hypokalemia*

- *Medications such as sodium bicarbonate and corticosteroids*

- *Nasogastric suctioning*

- *Diarrhea*

When interpreting primary acid-base disturbances, it is recommended that the acid-base status is interpreted first. Knowing that the normal pH is from 7.35-7.45, a pH of less than <7.35 is considered acidosis; and a pH >7.45 is considered alkalosis. The next step is to analyze the PaCO2. If the pH was normal and the PaCO2 is also within normal limits, then the acid-base balance is also considered normal; however, when the pH is low or high, the PaCO2 must be further explored. A pH that is low can indicate either respiratory or metabolic acidosis; a high pH can indicate either respiratory or metabolic alkalosis.

INBORN ERRORS OF METABOLISM

Inborn errors of metabolism are inherited genetic disorders caused by abnormal gene mutations. Most states have mandatory neonate testing for some of these disorders such as phenylketonuria, homocystinuria, maple syrup urine disease, tyrosinemia, biotinidase deficiency and galactosemia.

These inborn errors of metabolism are classified as disorders of:

- *Amino acids and organic acids*
- *Carbohydrates*
- *Fatty acids and glycerol*
- *Lysosomal storage*
- *Mitochondrial oxidative phosphorylation*
- *Purines and pyrimidine*

AMINO ACID AND ORGANIC ACID METABOLIC DISORDERS

Amino acid and organic acid metabolic disorders include, among many others:

- *Phenylketonuria (PKU)*
- *Tyrosinemia*
- *Maple syrup urine disease, or branched-chain ketoaciduria*
- *Disorders of methionine metabolism*
- *Dihydropteridine reductase deficiency*
- *Pterin-4a-carbinolamine dehydratase deficiency*
- *Biopterin synthesis deficiency*
- *Propionic acidemia*
- *Multiple carboxylase deficiency*
- *Methylmalonic acidemia*

The first four of the above listed disorders are discussed below.

Phenylketonuria (PKU)

Phenylketonuria (PKU, which occurs most often among the white population, is characterized by a buildup of dietary phenylalanine, particularly in the brain, because dietary phenylalanine is not converted to tyrosine as it normally should be. Excesses can also be deposited into the urine for detection among neonates. This metabolic disorder is associated with profound deficits of intellectual and brain functioning.

Upon birth, most neonates appear asymptomatic; however, after several months the infant may show signs of hyperactivity, an eczema-type rash and an unusual odor of the urine and perspiration. During childhood years, the signs and symptoms can also include seizures, psychosis and disturbances of gait. The diagnosis is made with routine neonatal screening and phenylalanine levels.

All complications and manifestations of this metabolic disorder can be prevented with treatment during the early days of life; treatment after 2-3 years does not resolve some of these like seizures and hyperactivity. Infants and children have to be maintained on a life time of dietary phenylalanine restriction, therefore proteins (all of which contain phenylalanine) are limited. Other treatments include tyrosine supplementation, sapropterin, protein hydrolysates to remove phenylalanine and phenylalanine-free elemental amino acid mixtures.

Plasma phenylalanine levels are monitored and maintained between 2 mg/dL and 4 mg/dL when the child is less than 12 years of age and between 2 mg/dL and 10 mg/dL for children older than 12 years of age.

Tyrosine Metabolism Disorders

Tyrosine is the precursor of hormone, melanin and neurotransmitters such as norepinephrine, epinephrine and dopamine. Newborns can be affected with a transient and temporary form of tyrosinemia which can also be detected, like PKU, with routine neonatal screening.

Some infants are asymptomatic and others have signs and symptoms such as poor feeding and lethargy. It is diagnosed with elevated plasma tyrosine levels.

In addition to transient neonatal tyrosinemia, there are other types of tyrosinemia, including Type I, II and III.

Maple Syrup Urine Disease (Branched-chain Ketoaciduria)

Maple syrup urine disease, a type of branched-chain ketoaciduria, can lead to severe metabolic acidosis as the result of a collection of organic acids secondary to the autosomal, recessive lack of enzymes. The clinical signs and symptoms include the characteristic odor of maple syrup bodily odor, particularly in the cerumen, as well as perinatal illnesses, lethargy, vomiting, seizures, coma and death when it is not promptly diagnosed and treated. The patient is adversely affected with academia and ketonemia.

The diagnosis is made when laboratory blood tests reveal elevated plasma levels of these branched chain amino acids, especially leucine.

Some of the treatments include hemodialysis, peritoneal dialysis, dietary restrictions of branched-chain amino acids, fluid hydration, high dose thiamin of about 200 mg orally every 24 hours and high dose dextrose. A liver transplantation provides the cure.

Disorders of Methionine Metabolism

These disorders adversely affect clotting, the skeletal system and the CNS. For example, these disorders place the affected patient at risk for thrombosis and abnormalities of the brain and spinal cord including intellectual dysfunction. Classical excesses of homocysteine lead to thrombosis as well as adverse skeletal and neurological system effects.

The diagnosis is made with neonatal screening that detects elevated total plasma homocysteine and serum methionine.

The treatment of this neonatal error of metabolism is high doses of pyridoxine with a dosage of 100 to 500 mg orally every 24 hours, a low methionine diet, trimethylglycine at a dosage of 100 to 125 mg/kg orally two times a day to increase remethylation and to lower homocysteine, as well as 500 to 1000 µg of folate once daily.

CARBOHYDRATE METABOLIC DISORDERS

There are several broad categories of carbohydrate errors of metabolism including, among many others, glycogen storage disorders like galactosemia. Glycogen storage disorders impede glycogen breakdown or synthesis from the liver or the muscles, thus causing hypoglycemia or the collection of abnormal amounts of glycogen in the tissues of the body.

Generally speaking, the signs and symptoms of these disorders are myopathy and hypoglycemia, and they are diagnosed when an MRI or biopsy detects glycogen in the tissues and there is a decrease of liver and muscle functioning in terms of enzyme activity.

Treatments include dietary supplementation of cornstarch to sustain and maintain glucose when the liver is the source of the problem and exercise avoidance with the muscular forms of this disorder.

Galactosemia

This enzyme deficiency prevents the conversion of galactose to glucose.

The signs and symptoms include renal dysfunction, liver failure and cognitive deficits. It is diagnosed with laboratory red blood cell enzyme analysis.

The treatment consists of the dietary elimination of galactose, which is found in fruits, vegetables and dairy products.

Diabetic Ketoacidosis

Diabetic ketoacidosis occurs as the result of severe hyperglycemia over 300 mg/dL and a severe life threatening, emergency situation. Pathophysiological characterization of diabetic ketoacidosis includes the presence of ketones in the urine and blood, as well as the breakdown of bodily fat for energy. The onset is very rapid; it is associated with a high rate of mortality when left untreated. Diabetic ketoacidosis can occur as the result of trauma, insufficient insulin and the poor management of a co-existing acute disease or disorder.

The signs and symptoms of diabetic ketoacidosis usually develop rapidly and include nausea and vomiting, abdominal pain, confusion, excessive thirst, weakness or fatigue, shortness of breath, fruity-scented breath, the presence of ketones in the urine and blood, dyspnea, dehydration, electrolyte imbalances, frequent urination and coma.

Patients diagnosed with diabetic ketoacidosis may be treated in the emergency department or may have to be admitted to the hospital for treatment. Treatment includes a three-step process, which includes rapid rehydration with an isotonic fluid like 0.9% sodium chloride followed with infusions of hypotonic 0.45% sodium chloride, replacement of electrolytes like sodium, chloride and potassium, insulin therapy intravenously until the blood glucose is less than 240 mg/dL and no longer acidic, and the administration of sodium bicarbonate slowly via the intravenous route when the pH is less than 7.0. If diabetic ketoacidosis is not treated the patient risks unconsciousness and death.

GASTROINTESTINAL DISORDERS

The patient's physical status and condition is also impacted by a number of different gastrointestinal diseases and disorders such as:

- *Congenital anomalies*
- *Abdominal distension*
- *Feeding tube placement*
- *Necrotizing enterocolitis*

Gastrointestinal Congenital Anomalies

Some of the most commonly occurring gastrointestinal congenital anomalies include:

- *Meconium ileus*
- *Meconium plug syndrome*

Meconium Ileus

Meconium ileus is present when thick and tenacious meconium obstructs the terminal ileum causing a small bowel obstruction; micro-colon, an abnormally narrow portion of the colon, occurs distal to the obstruction. Some of the complications of this disorder include mal-rotation and twisting of the bowel, intestinal atresia, perforation, respiratory distress, ascites, intestinal infarcts, intestinal atresia and sterile meconium peritonitis.

The signs and symptoms of meconium ileus include abdominal distension, vomiting, a failure to pass meconium within 24 hours after birth and palpable distended small bowel loops. The diagnosis is made with x-rays, a barium enema and a positive test for cystic fibrosis.

Less complicated cases can be treated with an enema with a radiographic contrast medium and N-acetyl cysteine; when unsuccessful, a double barreled ileostomy is performed and N-acetyl cysteine lavages evacuate the meconium.

Meconium Plug Syndrome of the Small Left Colon

This disorder can occur among healthy infants, however, it is most commonly found among infants of mothers who have had diabetes and/or toxemia with magnesium sulfate treatments during pregnancy. This syndrome reflects a functional immaturity of the colon.

The signs and symptoms include the infant's inability to defecate, abdominal distention, vomiting and sometimes a complete gastrointestinal obstruction. The diagnosis of meconium plug syndrome is done with x-rays, a contrast enema and sometimes testing to rule out Hirschsprung's disease.

Water soluble contrast enemas to expel the plug from the intestinal wall and surgical decompression may be indicated.

Abdominal Distention

Abdominal distension is a symptom rather than a disorder. Abdominal distention occurs when a gas or fluid collects in the abdominal space. Some of the underlying causes of abdominal distention include:

- *Celiac disease*
- *Liver disease*
- *Cardiac disease*
- *Infections such as hookworm and other parasitic infections*

- *Diverticulitis*
- *Bowel obstruction*
- *Lactose intolerance*
- *Inflammatory bowel disease like irritable bowel syndrome and Crohn's disease*

The signs and symptoms can include distention and expansion of the stomach, feelings of fullness and bloating, pain, cramping and shortness of breath when the distention creates pressure on the diaphragm and lungs.

The treatment aims to correct the underlying disorder. Over-the-counter medications to relieve gas can also be recommended.

Malabsorption

Malabsorption is a gastrointestinal disorder characterized by the lack of ability to absorb one or more nutrients. Malabsorption can be categorized as occurring from primary or secondary causes; some primary causes are celiac disease and lactose intolerance and some secondary causes include pancreatic disease, a gastric bypass and inflammatory bowel disease.

This gastrointestinal disorder can adversely affect the absorption of protein, carbohydrates or fat. Fat malabsorption is the most common, and, because vitamins A, D, E and K are fat-soluble, the absorption of these vitamins is impaired when a person has impaired fat absorption. The complications include malnutrition and fluid and electrolyte imbalances.

The signs and symptoms vary according to the specific nutrient that is not absorbed. Steatorrhea (fatty stools,) flatulence, abdominal distention and loud bowel sounds, referred to as borborygmi, are signs of fat malabsorption. Abdominal bloating and cramping are signs of altered carbohydrate absorption; muscular tenderness and the loss of muscle mass are signs of protein malabsorption. The diagnosis is made with a complete history and physical examination as well as radiographic and laboratory studies as based on the specific disorder and its underlying cause.

The treatment depends on the disorder. For example, celiac disease is treated by eliminating gluten from the diet; lactase intolerance is treated with dietary restrictions of milk products as well as dietary enzyme supplementation.

FEEDING TUBE PLACEMENT

Enteral nutrition is the administration of nutrients directly into the gastrointestinal tract with a tube feeding. Nasogastric tube feedings are preferred over gastrostomy tubes among patients who have intact swallowing and gag reflexes and lower esophageal sphincter control to prevent reflux. A percutaneous endoscopic gastrostomy (PEG) tube is used when long term enteral nutrition is needed. This tube is endoscopically placed through the abdominal wall into the stomach with a local anesthetic.

Enteral feedings can be administered on a continuous basis, intermittently or as a bolus. The procedure for the administration of an enteral feeding is below.

1. A high Fowler's position or at least a 30 degree angle is necessary

2. Verification of NG tube placement is done by measuring the length of the tube from the nose, and injecting 10 to 30 mL of air while auscultating over the upper left quadrant

3. Flush the tube with 30 to 50 mL of water before and after the feeding or every 4 to 6 hours when a continuous feeding is being given

4. Some of the complications of enteral tube feedings include diarrhea, particularly when a high caloric density formula is used, tube blockage, bacterial contamination, aspiration and regurgitation.

Necrotizing Enterocolitis

Necrotizing enterocolitis primarily affects premature infants. This disorder, the most common gastrointestinal emergency among neonates, leads to intestinal necrosis. Some of the risk factors associated with necrotizing enterocolitis include enteral tube feedings, prolonged rupture of the membranes, prematurity, congenital heart disease and infant feedings with hypertonic formulas.

It is possible the risk for this disorder can be decreased by providing TPN instead of oral feedings among neonates who are premature or very ill. It is also believed that breast milk, rather than formula feedings, and the administration of probiotics can decrease the risk. In order for this disorder to occur, three intestinal factors are typically present. These include:

- Preceding ischemic damage
- Colonization with bacteria
- Some intraluminal substance like an enteral feeding

Necrosis begins in the mucosa and later it can spread and involve the full thickness of the intestinal wall. This necrosis can lead to perforation, peritonitis, free floating air in the abdomen, sepsis and death.

The presenting signs and symptoms include lethargy, apnea, metabolic acidosis, signs of sepsis, abdominal distension, redness of the abdominal wall, rectal bleeding emesis, poor feeding, bloody stool, instability of the bodily temperature and bloating. The diagnosis is made with abdominal x-rays and laboratory studies that reveal neutropenia, thrombocytopenia and metabolic acidosis.

The treatments, depending on the severity, include parenteral fluids, the cessation of any tube feedings, nasogastric suction, TPN up to 21 days at times, antibiotics, special precaution isolation and a surgical resection of the stricture that most often occurs in the left colon; an ostomy is often necessary. Surgical interventions are necessary when the infant has signs of peritonitis or an intestinal perforation, also referred to as a pneumoperitoneum.

MUSCULOSKELETAL DISORDERS

A number of musculoskeletal disorders can also impact on the patient's respiratory status. Some of these musculoskeletal disorders include:

- *Spinal cord injuries*
- *Myopathies*
- *Spina bifida and myelomeningocele*
- *SMA*
- *Scolisosis*
- *Myelomeningocele*

Spinal Cord Injuries

Spinal cord injuries are frequently encountered in the emergency department. According to the American Spinal Injury Association, injuries can be classified from Grades A to E according to motor and sensory deficits.

A. *Complete.* The most severe grade of injury, with no sensory or motor function.

B. *Sensory Incomplete.* Characterized by a lack of sensory function at the level of the injury and below and a lack of motor function three levels below the motor level on both of the body's sides.

C. *Motor Incomplete.* Characterized by motor function preserved below the neurological level (such as with voluntary anal sphincter contraction) and more than half of key muscle functions affected by some level of paraplegia.

D. *Motor Incomplete.* Characterized by motor function preserved below the neurological level and less than half of key muscle functions are affected by some level of paralysis.

E. *Normal.* Sensory and motor function are normal, regardless of prior deficits.

Spinal cord injuries are also categorized as tetraplegia and paraplegia injuries. Tetraplegia is the loss, or impairment of, sensory and/or motor function originating at the cervical portion of the spinal cord; this type of injury causes absent or diminished functioning of the trunk, pelvic organs arms and legs. Paraplegia is the loss, or diminished functioning, of sensory and/or motor function from the thoracic, lumbar or sacral portion of the spinal cord. This type of injury causes impaired functioning of the pelvic organs, trunk, and legs without any arm involvement.

Spinal cord injuries are also categorized according to types of force exerted to produce it. These include flexion, extension, compression and rotation.

Flexion motion injuries, or burst fractures, most commonly occur with a car accident when the neck is hyper-flexed as the victim's chin is forcefully moved onto the chest; it dislocates the spine and ruptures the posterior ligaments. Extension injuries, referred to as hangman's fractures, occur when the head is tossed backwards; it fractures the posterior aspects of the vertebral body and ruptures the anterior ligament.

Compression injuries, or axial load injuries, can result from a dive into shallow water or a serious fall; the vertebral bodies become compressed and wedged and bone shards pierce the spinal cord. Rotational injuries can occur as the result of a variety of injuries and they are the most unstable of all flexion rotation injuries; these injuries damage the entire ligamentous structure.

Lastly, spinal cord injuries can be classified as penetrating and non-penetrating. All spinal cord injuries, except those that result from a gunshot or knife stabbing wound, are considered non-penetrating. Penetrating spinal cord injuries are serious and unstable.

The signs and symptoms of spinal cord injuries vary, as discussed above, according to the type of injury and the extent of the injury. In addition to the previously discussed signs and symptoms, other signs that occur as the result of spinal cord injuries include the compromise of the ABCs, impaired vital lung capacity, aspiration, hypoxia, impaired gas exchange, and diminished respiratory muscle function, all of which can lead to death when not treated.

Other possible signs and symptoms include pain, nausea, vomiting, impaired urinary function, paralytic ileus, and hypothermia, in addition to motor and sensory impairments including paralysis.

After the most severe and life threatening conditions are treated, further assessments are done as the nurse ensures that no flexion, extension or rotation of the patient's spine occurs. Log rolling and careful clothing removal are done to ensure spine stability.

Some of the commonly occurring complications of spinal cord injury include neurogenic shock, spinal shock, poikilothermia and autonomic dysreflexia.

Neurogenic shock, most often the result of a spinal cord injury at or below the T6 level, can lead to some life threatening complications like massive vasodilation, diminished venous return, alterations of tissue perfusion and decreased cardiac output. Neurogenic shock is characterized by hypotension as the result of peripheral vasodilation, the loss of sweating below the injury, hypothermia as the result of impaired sympathetic nervous system functioning, altered hypothalamus functioning, hypotension and bradycardia.

Spinal shock, which can persist for weeks after a cervical or upper thoracic spinal cord injury, can lead to a sudden loss of functioning below the level of the injury and other symptoms like flaccid paralysis of the bowel and bladder as well as priapism.

Poikilothermia, the body's loss of ability to control and regulate body temperature, is most commonly associated with injuries at and above T6. It is signaled with sweating and shivering, so it is important that body temperature is monitored and environmental temperature is controlled.

Autonomic dysreflexia, a life threatening condition, also occurs among patients with a spinal cord injury at or above T6. Autonomic dysreflexia is precipitated with bowel or bladder distention renal stones, tight clothing, a urinary tract infection, fractures, and hemorrhoids.

Some of the signs and symptoms of autonomic dysreflexia are significantly high blood pressure, headache, paleness and pallor, shortness of breath, anxiety, blurry vision and compensatory bradycardia.

Treatment goals include the identification and elimination of the precipitating cause and the use of nitrates or nifedipine. To treat, the spine is kept in neutral alignment and immobilized at all times with the exception of when the airway has to be opened to sustain life. A Kendrick Extrication Device, used in addition to a cervical collar, sandbags or commercially available head restraints are used to immobilize a patient's head, neck and spine in the normal anatomical, or neutral, position.

Severe to moderate pain is treated with morphine or fentanyl. Anticonvulsants, tricyclic antidepressants, anti-emetics and a nasogastric tube for distention, the prevention of a paralytic ileus, nausea and vomiting, as well as intubation and mechanical intervention are often indicated. Prophylactic anticoagulant therapy with low-molecular-weight heparin or low-dose heparin, compression stockings and intermittent sequential calf-compression devices are used to prevent deep vein thrombosis. A urinary catheter is used to treat a-contractile neuropathic bladder and to ensure adequate urinary output. Intake and output are monitored and accurately documented.

Spina Bifida

Spina bifida is a neural tube defect that is characterized by a failure of the vertebral column to close. It appears that low maternal folate levels may be a cause in addition to other factors such as genetics, maternal diabetes and some medications such as valproate. It can be suspected in utero with an ultrasonography and with elevated maternal α-fetoprotein and/or the presence of large amounts of amniotic fluids. This defect can vary greatly. Spina bifida can be occult with no signs of an anomaly or neurological deficits and it can also have a sac, which is referred to as spina bifida cystic, or even more severe as an open spine, referred to as rachischisis, with significant neurological losses and dysfunction distal to the deformity and the risk of mortality.

Some of the signs and symptoms are hydrocephalus, neurological deficits such as sensory losses and paralysis, muscular atrophy, loss of bladder and rectal sphincter control, neurogenic bladder, hydronephrosis, kyphosis, kidney damage and signs of hydrocephalus including increased intracranial pressure, apnea, stridor and swallowing problems.

Depending on the severity of this deformity, some of the treatment options include surgical repair of the lesion, a ventricular shunt to relieve the hydrocephalus and other urological and orthopedic corrections as indicated.

Myelomeningocele

Myelomeningocele is immediately covered with a sterile dressing after birth; prophylactic antibiotics are administered when the myelomeningocele is leaking in order to prevent meningitis. Surgical repair of a myelomeningocele and open forms of spina bifida are surgically repaired within 72 hours after birth.

SMA (Spinal Muscular Atrophy)

SMAs are a constellation of genetic disorders typified by progressive skeletal muscle wasting and degeneration. The types are as follows:

- Known as Werdnig-Hoffmann disease; characterized by hypotonia, highly pronounced problems with breathing, eating and sucking. Respiratory failure and death often occurs during the first year of life.

- Flaccid muscles, muscular weakness and fasciculations, dysphagia, absent deep tendon reflexes. Usually fetal as the result of respiratory failure; some children spontaneously stop progressing but retain damage that occurred prior to recovery.

- Known as Wohlfart-Kugelberg-Welander disease, Type III SMA is similar to Type I, but the child's life expectancy is longer and the progression is slower. Some may have a normal life span. Muscular wasting and weakness marches from proximal to distal areas and usually begins in the hips and the quadriceps.

- Type IV may not appear until the person is 30-60 years of age. It progresses slowly and often affects only proximal muscles. It somewhat mimics amyotrophic lateral sclerosis.

The diagnosis is made based on genetic composition and testing such as electromyography and nerve conduction studies.

Treatment is supportive and it can consist of physical therapy, braces, and adaptive devices to facilitate daily living activities.

Myopathies: MD (Muscular Dystrophy)

MD is a progressive, inherited disorder that affects muscular function and structure. There are several types of MD, of which Duchenne's is the most severe and the most common. This form is quite similar to Becker MD, except that Becker is not as severe and it has a later onset. Other forms include:

- *Emery-Dreifuss dystrophy*
- *Myotonic dystrophy*
- *Limb-girdle dystrophy*
- *Facioscapulohumeral*

The signs and symptoms, which typically emerge when the child is 2 to 3 years of age include progressive weakness of the muscles of the legs, initially, unsteady gait, frequent falls, flexion contractures, pseudo-hypertrophy of the calves, respiratory compromise, cardiac muscle abnormities like arrhythmias, conduction dysfunction and cardiomyopathy.

The diagnosis is confirmed with an immunostained analysis of dystrophin obtained with a biopsy and DNA mutation testing.

The treatment aims to improve the quality and the quantity of life. Some of these interventions include supportive care, prednisone, physical therapy, corrective surgery, leg braces and the administration of a β-blocker or an ACE inhibitor for cardiac problems. Respiratory support measures range from noninvasive ventilator support to a tracheotomy and ventilation, as indicated.

Scoliosis

Scoliosis, a curvature of the spine, is most often discovered when children are between 10 and 16 years of age.

The signs and symptoms of scoliosis can include complaints of back pain, a leg-length discrepancy and asymmetry of the chest wall. An x-ray of the spine confirms the diagnosis. Curves more than 10° are considered significant.

Depending on the severity, some treatments include physical therapy, braces, and spinal fusion with rod placement for severe cases.

ANTICIPATING CARE BASED ON LABORATORY RESULTS AND NUTRITIONAL STATUS

Respiratory therapists continuously monitor a wide variety of hematologic, chemistry, microbiological laboratory studies in addition to other quantitative data such as blood gas analysis, co-oximetry and any complications of feedings that can indicate an abnormal finding or event that necessitates the intervention(s) of the respiratory therapist.

NORMAL VALUES

Normal values for any laboratory tests not previously covered, as well as normal blood gas analysis and co-oximetry tests, are discussed below. All abnormal values have implications for the RT's ability to anticipate care.

CHEMISTRY LABORATORY TESTS

Albumin

The normal range of albumin is 3.4 - 5.4 g/dL. Low albumin is a sign of renal and/or hepatic disease such as hepatitis, cirrhosis and malabsorption. Elevated albumin levels can indicate dehydration.

MICROBIOLOGY TESTS

Some of the microbiology tests that respiratory therapists most closely monitor include those for:

- *RSV swabs*
- *Gram staining*
- *Cultures and sensitivities*

RSV (Respiratory Syncytial Virus) Swabs

RSV swabs are done in order to differentiate this virus from the common cold or another infection particularly when the patient is compromised with a chronic disorder or another acute illness. The sample is obtained by using a cotton swab or a nasal wash to collect nasal drainage.

COMPLICATIONS OF FEEDINGS

Neonatal feeding and nutrition problems can occur as the result of those listed below, among others.

- *Feeding intolerance*

- *Aspiration*

- *Misplacement of a feeding tube*

Feeding Intolerance

Feeding intolerance is a risk for low weight, preterm neonates and one of the leading causes of growth and development failures. It also places the infant at risk for infection and long term neurological and cognitive deficits. It appears that low weight neonates are affected with this disorder because they have less motility, absorption and intestinal length than full term infants.

Some of the signs, symptoms and complications of this disorder include abdominal distention, gastric residual, emesis, bloody stools, bowel edema and even life-threatening necrotizing enterocolitis. Some of the respiratory and cardiovascular-related signs and symptoms include:

- *Apnea*

- *Bradycardia*

- *An unstable bodily temperature instability*

- *Hypotension*

The treatment goal is to establish and maintain adequate nutrition. Enteral tube feedings, as previously discussed, are given.

MISPLACEMENT OF A FEEDING TUBE

A misplacement of a feeding tube is particularly common among young children. When these tubes are misplaced, aspiration is a real risk. Patients receiving tube feedings should be maintained at least at a 30 degree angle and the nurses must check the placement of the feeding tube before administering any feedings. This verification of NG tube placement is done injecting 10 to 30 mL of air while auscultating over the upper left quadrant

THE EFFECTS OF PHARMACOLOGIC AGENTS

As previously discussed, medications have both desirable and undesirable effects, as well as adverse reactions. Although RTs do not administer many of these medications, they must have applicable knowledge of medication effects, side effects and adverse reactions as they monitor patients, alongside the skills necessary to anticipate these effects. Some medications that RTs must thoroughly understand include:

- *Sedatives and hypnotics*

- *Analgesia*

- *Neuromuscular blocking agents like succinylcholine and cisatracurium*

- *Antibiotics*

- *Mucolytic medications*

- *Leukotriene Modifiers*

- *Bronchodilators*

- *Anti-inflammatory medications*

- *Corticosteroids*

- *Vasodilators*

Sedatives and Hypnotics

- Desired Effect(s): Sedation for sleep, decreased anxiety and pre-anesthesia

- Side Effects: Tolerance, respiratory system depression, REM rebound and dependence

- Adverse Reactions: Respiratory distress and laryngospasm

Analgesia

- Desired Effect(s): The relief of pain

- Side Effects of NSAIDS: Gastrointestinal bleeding, ulcers, fluid retention, hypertension, renal problems, cardiac problems and rashes.

- Side Effects of Opioid Analgesic Agents: Respiratory depression, constipation, lethargy and dependence

- Adverse Reactions: Respiratory arrest

Neuromuscular Blocking Agents

- Desired Effect(s): To eliminate spontaneous breathing, to facilitate tracheal intubation, to decrease oxygen consumption among mechanically ventilated patients, and to minimize higher dosages of anesthetic agents for muscle relaxation.
- Side Effects: Allergic reaction, tachycardia bronchospasm
- Adverse Reactions: Circulatory collapse

Antibiotics

- Desired Effect(s): To treat infections and act as prophylaxis against infection
- Side Effects: Super-infections, sensitivity,
- Adverse Reactions: Organ toxicity and anaphylactic shock

Mucolytic Medications

- Desired Effect(s): To thin, loosen and expel respiratory secretions
- Side Effects: Skin rash, fever, clammy skin and increased lung secretions
- Adverse Reactions: None known

Leukotriene Modifiers

- Desired Effect(s): Inhibits bronchoconstriction and smooth muscle contractions
- Side Effects: Headache, fatigue, nasal congestion, cough, dyspepsia and abdominal pain
- Adverse Reactions: None known

Bronchodilators

- Desired Effect(s): Dilation of the bronchioles and bronchi, increased airflow and decreased resistance

- Side Effects: Nausea, vomiting, diarrhea, headache, rapid or irregular heartbeat, muscle cramps, nervousness, palpitations and hyperactivity.

- Adverse Reactions: Paradoxical bronchial constriction, cardiac arrhythmias, cardiac arrest and hypertension.

Anti-inflammatory Medications

- Desired Effect(s): Decrease inflammation, body temperature and pain

- Side Effects: Diarrhea, hearing loss, rash, heartburn and confusion

- Adverse Reactions: Tinnitus, agranulocytosis, anaphylaxis and blood dyscrasias

Vasodilators

- Desired Effect(s): Decrease blood pressure

- Side Effects: Dizziness, vertigo, tinnitus, headache, urinary frequency and dry mouth

- Adverse Reactions: Pancreatitis, orthostatic hypotension, tachycardia and palpitations

END-OF-LIFE CARE

Death is a process. Patients die from:

- A brief, steady decline, like many affected with cancer

- A long, slow decline, like many with chronic illness and events like cerebrovascular disease;

- A quick process resulting in death, as from an acute episode or exacerbation of an existing disease such a sudden acute myocardial infarction or death from heart failure.

It is less complicated and challenging to determine life expectancy and the time of death among those who have a brief, steady decline than it is among those who have a prolonged chronic disorder. When a patient is potentially dying, they should be given complete information and the opportunity to discuss their care goals and make decisions about many things including financial issues, family issues, final wishes and whether or not to undergo medical treatments or elect to choose palliative and hospice care.

Much of the information in this section does not apply to neonates. However, many concepts related to end-of-life care have broad applicability for family members – especially the parents – of neonatal patients at the end of their lives. As concepts related to end-of-life care are required knowledge for RTs, though not necessarily specific to neonatal care, they may appear on the NPS credentialing examination.

PALLIATIVE AND HOSPICE CARE

Palliative (curative) and hospice are two different philosophies or approaches to patient care. Hospice care aims to provide the patient and family members with comfort and support, rather than treatments to prolong life. The decision to forgo treatments and enter into hospice care is a personal decision and not encouraged or discouraged by the healthcare provider. Instead, the patient and family members should learn about hospice care and its benefits in an objective manner without coercion so they can make a knowledgeable decision. Hospice care, as a philosophy, can be rendered in all settings including a free standing hospice center in the community, a medical center, long term care facility and in the home.

WITHDRAWAL OF LIFE SUPPORT

The withdrawal of life support is defined as withdrawal of ventilator support, with or without extubation, and withdrawal or foregoing of additional life sustaining treatments like cardiopulmonary resuscitation, vasopressors, blood products, hemodialysis, nutrition, and antibiotics, thus allowing a natural death to occur from the patient's underlying disease process. This decision should be made in collaboration with the patient or the health care surrogate unless the withdrawal was previously documented in an advance directive.

Although procedures vary according to the specific healthcare facility, most include the use of sedation, the gradual or abrupt cessation of mechanical ventilation/extubation by the respiratory therapist, ordered medications that are given even when they may hasten death, and the monitoring and treatment of any distress or discomfort that can be manifested with the use of accessory muscles, agitation, grimacing, tachycardia, hypertension, tachypnea over 35 respirations per minute, gasping and noisy respirations.

CARING FOR ORGAN DONORS

The U.S. Department of Health and Human Services' document, *Critical Pathway for the Organ Donor (Appendix 3)* [12] outlines the necessary care for organ donors. It can be accessed at the provided URL.

---

[12] https://www.unos.org/docs/Critical_Pathway.pdf

PERIDEATH

The perideath ("around death") experience consists of preparation, death itself and the third phase, which is after death. Some of the signs and symptoms that occur in preparation for death include:

- *Bodily coolness*
- *Excessive sleeping*
- *Decreases of food and fluids*
- *Incontinence*
- *Congestion*
- *Changes in breathing patterns, like Cheyne-Stokes respirations*

- *Disorientation*
- *Restlessness*
- *Withdrawal*
- *Vision-like experiences*
- *Letting go*
- *Saying goodbye*

PSYCHOSOCIAL, EMOTIONAL AND SPIRITUAL ISSUES

Some of the most commonly occurring psychological and emotional alterations associated with terminal disease include anger, denial, grief and loss, fear and anxiety, guilt, depression, suicidal and homicidal ideation, loss of hope and meaning, sleep disturbances, alterations of bodily image, loss of control, poor coping, intimacy and relationship issues and nearing death awareness.

ANGER AND ANXIETY

Anger

Many patients in pain and/or at the end of life experience anger and hostility. Patient's family members and significant others may also experience these same feelings. Anger is a common psychological response to these conditions, as described below in the Kubler-Ross Stages of Grieving model.

Simply defined, anger is a psychological or emotional state that is related to displeasure. It is often accompanied with feelings of guilt because it is not socially acceptable to be angry and to express these feelings. Outward expressions of anger can include hostility toward others, destructiveness, aggression and even violence. At times, anger can be directed toward the precipitating event, and at other times it is displaced toward others when employing the psychological defense mechanism of displacement. For example, a patient becomes angry about their loss of independence and functioning as a result of their illness, then directs (displaces) this anger towards their spouse, family members, nurse and other members of the healthcare team.

Healthcare providers can intervene in terms of anger and hostility by accepting the fact that the patient has the right to be angry and attempt to understand the meaning and the source of the anger, as well as to encourage the patient to openly ventilate their anger.

Anxiety

Anxiety is accompanied with feelings of dread, discomfort, and apprehension. It leads to autonomic responses and the anticipation of danger.

Anxiety can be categorized as mild, moderate, severe and panic level. Death anxiety commonly affects those with terminal illnesses; it is characterized by various degrees of dread and discomfort. The patient may express fears about the events surrounding death like incontinence and the loss of cognitive abilities, pain at the time of death, uncertainty regarding a higher power, and fears about the impact of their death on family members, among other things.

The signs and symptoms of anxiety include affective (increased helplessness, irritability, fright and worry), behavioral (insomnia and vigilance), sympathetic (anorexia, increased pulse, blood pressure and pulse), physiological (diaphoresis and trembling), parasympathetic (fatigue, urinary changes, weakness and faintness) and cognitive (poor problem solving and a lack of attention span.)

Respiratory therapists should assess the level of anxiety for both the patient and the significant other. As based on this assessment, some of the treatment interventions can include empathy when the anxiety is rational, encouraging the person to ventilate their feelings and perceptions, explaining all procedures, and using some techniques like relaxation, positive self-talk, massage and therapeutic touch.

DEFENSE MECHANISMS

There are many psychological (or ego) defense mechanisms. These are unconscious processes that protect the patient from the stress that arises with inner tensions and conflicts. Defense mechanisms are the precursor to coping in a cognitive, conscious manner.

Denial

- Mechanism: The patient refuses to acknowledge facts or realities that are threatening to them.

- Protective Purpose: Stops the person from being adversely affected by a traumatic event or reality until they are ready to do so.

- Example: A patient is diagnosed with a disease like lung cancer or HIV/AIDS and refuses to change their lifestyle or accept treatment because they don't believe the diagnosis.

Reaction Formation

- Mechanism: The person acts in a manner opposite to their true feelings.

- Protective Purpose: Allows the person to act out their feelings in a more appropriate manner.

- Example: A woman resents her husband, but vocally supports all of their ideas and suggestions in a cooperative and polite manner.

Sublimation

- Mechanism: An unacceptable sexual or aggressive urge is replaced with a socially acceptable activity that substitutes for it.

- Protective Purpose: Protects the person from acting in a socially unacceptable, impulsive manner.

- Example: A person with incestuous feelings may become active in community service.

Undoing

- Mechanism: Acting in a manner that "makes up for" or atones for wrongdoing.

- Protective Purpose: Allows the person to rid themselves of guilt.

- Example: An abusive husband brings flowers home to his wife.

Compensation

- Mechanism: Personal weakness is covered up with overachievement in another area.

- Protective Purpose: Allows the person to protect their ego and level of self-esteem by excelling in another area to make up for their weakness.

- Example: A dyslexic child with an older sibling who excels in school may choose to become a piano virtuoso to make up for scholastic weaknesses.

Displacement

- Mechanism: Displacement moves hostility from one person or object to another.

- Protective Purpose: Allows the affected individual to express their true feelings, but in a manner that is less harmful and dangerous.

- Example: A man who has been fired from work may come home and punch a hole in the wall, rather than punching the boss.

Projection

- Mechanism: Believing that other people or the environment are the factors that have led to the patient's weaknesses, shortcomings, and failures.

- Protective Purpose: Helps the patient to protect their own self-image and self-esteem by placing blame on other people or the environment.

- Example: A college student who fails out of college blames the college and the professors rather than him/herself.

Repression

- Mechanism: Repression helps the person to keep threatening thoughts, desires and feelings deep down so they do not erupt into consciousness.

- Protective Purpose: Protects the person from trauma until they are ready to cope and deal with it.

- Example: A patient may experience repressive amnesia after a traumatic automobile accident that does not allow them to remember any events surrounding and after the accident.

Regression

- Mechanism: Regression takes the person to a less demanding and threatening stage of development.

- Protective Purpose: Moves the person back to a previous stage of development when they were able to be cared for and dependent upon, others.

- Example: An ill hospitalized 8-year-old child may regress to thumb sucking and bed-wetting.

Identification

- Mechanism: The affected patient imitates the behaviors of a person that they fear.

- Protective Purpose: Helps the patient preserve the value of self and prevent personal devaluation.

- Example: A child imitates the father that she fears.

Minimization

- Mechanism: The affected patient minimizes the significance of a problem.

- Protective Purpose: Allows the person to avoid taking responsibility and accountability for their own actions.

- Example: A diabetic patient with severe leg ulcerations may state that it is "no big deal."

Rationalization

- Mechanism: Attaching socially acceptable motives and faulty logic to actions and behaviors.

- Protective Purpose: Helps the person to cope with their inability to meet standards and goals.

- Example: A husband who pushes his wife rationalizes it by stating that his wife was not hurt.

Introjection

- Mechanism: A person accepts norms, values and beliefs as one's own despite the fact that they are not consistent, and contrary to, those that the person previously held.

- Protective Purpose: Prevents the person from being ostracized by society.

- Example: A person may suddenly embark upon a healthy lifestyle and personal responsibility when, in the past, they did not.

Intellectualization

- Mechanism: Forced rational thinking is used to decrease the significance of a threatening and traumatic event.

- Protective Purpose: Protects the person from psychological trauma and pain.

- Example: The spouse of a diabetic who has died may state that her husband did not want to live with his complications of diabetes anyway.

Healthcare professionals should not strip these psychological mechanisms away from the patient. They should simply acknowledge the person and their feelings but NOT argue with the patient about their lack of insight or better coping mechanisms. These mechanisms are beneficial to the patient; they protect the person from psychological distress and other problems.

Depression

Depression, of varying degrees, often affects the patient and those close to the patient when the person is affected with a serious, terminal illness like cancer. Depression leads to physical, emotional and cognitive changes.

The signs and symptoms of depression include feelings of hopelessness, helplessness, sadness, dejection, despair, sleep loss, listlessness, headache, weight loss, anorexia, social withdrawal, lack of sexual desire, crying, poor levels of concentration, poor decision making and problem solving skills, diminished performance, personality changes, and a lack of self-worth and self-esteem.

The care and treatment for a depressed patient is multifaceted. The patient needs social support, perhaps spiritual support, cognitive behavioral therapy, medications such as antidepressants, and non-pharmacological approaches such as stress reduction and relaxation techniques. Medications are often a concern due to the fact that these medications may serve as the vehicle for a future suicide attempt.

Fear

Fear is a feeling of dread and apprehension relating to some impending danger or threat. It, too, can result from a real or unreal threat, but nonetheless, the patient is adversely affected with it. Although fear and anxiety are highly similar and often occurring simultaneously, they are also different. The source of fear is identifiable and the source of anxiety is often unidentifiable.

Some of the signs and symptoms include apprehension, muscular tension, feelings of dread, panic, terror, jitteriness, diminished cognitive and problem solving skills, dyspnea, dry mouth, fatigue, rapid pulse and respirations, increased systolic blood pressure, nausea, vomiting, pallor, pupil dilation, increased alertness with a narrowed focus on the source of the fear, avoidance and/or aggression.

Interventions, after assessment, can include confronting the fear, verbalizing the fearful feeling, assisting the patient to distinguish between real and imagined threats, and psychological support measures such as cognitive behavioral therapy, relaxation techniques and massage.

Distress

Distress can be described as troubling feelings in a patient that can range from mild to severe and even disabling. A patient can experience distress at any time from diagnosis and treatment to palliative care and can occur in different severities as a patient's disease or disorder progresses. It can impact their ability to be able to cope with all types of situations, and often times when a patient is in distress they are unable to deal with even the simplest of situations.

Distress can be seen with a variety of different physical, emotional, mental and behavioral symptoms, including back pain, headaches, anxiety, depression and moodiness.

Treatment for distress can be in the form of relaxation techniques, counseling, and educating the patient on hope and how effective that tool is. Patients in distress need the support of family, friends and healthcare personnel to overcome their feelings. Some of the symptoms can be treated with medications, both prescribed, such as antidepressants, benzodiazepines and pain medications, or non-prescribed, such as ibuprofen. Other tools, such as heating pads or ice packs, tens units etc. can also be helpful to alleviate some of the symptoms.

Guilt

Like all of the other psychosocial issues, the family and significant others are often affected with feelings of guilt and ambivalence. For example, the patient may experience feelings of guilt for the effect that their lung cancer is having on the family unit after years of the family's attempts to convince the patient to stop smoking. A patient may also feel guilty about leaving their family in poor financial status because of the medical expenses associated with the illness. Families may also experience feelings of guilt because they may have not cared for the person enough or they are no longer able to care for the palliative care patient.

The purpose of guilt is to alert the person that they have done something wrong. This feeling of guilt then encourages them to change their behavior so that it does not violate social and moral standards.

Some of the signs and symptoms associated with guilt can include physical, psychological and spiritual distress and despair. Healthcare professionals can teach the patient about the purpose of guilt in terms of learning and changing behavior, encouraging the patient to make amends, facilitating the patient's acceptance of the fact that they did something wrong but there is a need to move on and grow, and to understand that humans are not perfect and that forgiveness is possible.

Patients and family members may need psychological, spiritual and religious support to resolve feelings of guilt.

Loss of Hope and Meaning

The loss of hope can have psychological and spiritual or religious meanings and sources. For example, a person who is depressed may have feelings of hopelessness and no view of the future. The same patient may also experience spiritual loss of faith and hope. The meaning of life is also adversely affected with the presence of a serious illness. The concept, like hope, can also have psychological and well as spiritual and religious meaning. For example, a person may doubt the presence of an afterlife when they believed in it in the past.

A patient who is experiencing a loss of hope experiences the subjective state in which the person sees few or no alternatives and this leads to their inability to garner the energy and motivation to act on their own behalf.

Some of the signs and symptoms include decreased appetite, passivity, withdrawal, flat affect, withdrawal, a lack of involvement in care and the lack of motivation and initiative.

Some of the interventions for patients experiencing loss of hope and meaning include monitoring the patient for suicide risk, assisting the patient to discover sources of hope, assisting with problem solving, decision making, goal setting and coping, and encouraging the patient to verbalize their feelings in an open and trusting environment.

GRIEF AND LOSS

Loss, often associated with grief, is multidimensional. Loss can be actual, perceived, or anticipated. It occurs when a person has a significant change that causes the loss of something of value or when the person anticipates and/or perceived the loss of something of value.

Grieving is a normal response that includes physical, emotional, spiritual, social and intellectual responses. Sources of loss can originate from many things including a loss of self and one's bodily image because of the signs and symptoms of their cancer as well as surgical disfigurement, extra-personal losses like the loss of a home in a fire, and the loss of savings with a hospitalization and cancer care. All losses impact on the patient.

Perceived losses are those losses that are not verifiable by others. The patient with perceived loss experience feelings of grief because they perceive a loss that is not actually occurring. For example, an elderly woman may perceive that they are no longer useful to others, when in fact the woman is still actively engaging in social and charitable activities. This perception, although faulty, still impacts on and affects the person.

People have anticipatory grief and loss before an actual or perceived loss actually occurs. For example, a son may undergo severe anticipatory loss and grief soon after his mother has been diagnosed with terminal cancer. Similarly, a woman may have anticipatory loss relating to her their loss of sexuality after a mastectomy.

Theories and Conceptual Frameworks Relating to Grief and Loss

<u>Kubler Ross's Stages of Grieving</u>

Similar to the other theories of loss, grieving and death, Kubler Ross's stages of grieving include:

1. Denial
2. Anger
3. Bargaining
4. Depression
5. Acceptance

Bargaining is a unique phase of this theory. During the bargaining stage, the patient negotiates and bargains to avoid the loss. Spiritual support is often helpful during this stage.

<u>Engel's Stages of Grieving</u>

According to Engel, the stages of grieving are as below.

1. Shock and disbelief
2. Developing awareness
3. Restitution
4. Resolving the loss
5. Idealization
6. Outcome

During shock and disbelief the patient denies the loss and refuses to accept it. Later the patient consciously acknowledges the loss and may even express anger towards others including family members and healthcare professionals like the diabetes educator.

During the resolution stage, the patient contemplates the loss and may accept a dependent role in terms of their support network. Patients deify and idealize the lost loved one and may also experience guilt and ambivalence. During the outcome phase of Engel's model, the patient adjusts to the loss as based on their characteristics and the characteristics of the loss, as discussed above.

Sander's Phases of Bereavement

The phases of bereavement, according to Sander's theory, are:

1. *Shock*

2. *Awareness of the loss*

3. *Conservation and withdrawal*

4. *Healing- the turning point*

5. *Renewal*

These phases are quite similar to those of Engel with some variations. For example, during the conservation and withdrawal phase, the person will withdraw from others and attempt to restore their physical and emotional well-being; during the healing stage, the person will move from emotional distress to the point where they are able to learn how to live without the loved one. During the renewal phase, the person is able to independently live without the loved one.

The defining characteristics of grief can include sleep disturbances, altered immune responses, anger, blame, withdrawal, pain, panic, distress, suffering and alterations with neuroendocrine functioning.

We can assist the patient with the grieving process by encouraging the person to verbalize their feelings, encouraging effective coping strategies, involving the family and significant others in the care of the patient, and, when needed, referring the patient and significant others to sources of psychosocial and spiritual support.

DEATH AWARENESS

Patients and family members have one of three types of awareness. Levels of awareness impact on how the nurse communicates with these patients. The three types are closed awareness, mutual pretense and open awareness.

Closed awareness is defined as an awareness of impending death and terminal illness. Although not as often as was done in the past, some family members may choose to withhold complete and accurate information about the patient's condition from the patient affected with the illness. This poses ethical and communication challenges.

Mutual pretense is the type of awareness that is typified when the patient and significant others have an awareness of the patient's condition but all, including the patient, avoid all discussions about it. Mutual pretense leaves the affected patient with no one to talk to about their fears and concerns because the patient does not discuss things with the family and the family does not openly discuss things with the patient.

Open awareness is the most beneficial of all levels of awareness for the patient and their significant others. All know about the terminal nature of the disease and impending death and all are able to talk about it. Open awareness facilitates the patient's finalization of plans and affairs, such as funeral arrangements.

The signs, symptoms and patient/significant others' interactions depend on the level of awareness. For example, closed awareness is characterized by a lack of authentic communication and planning for the end of life; mutual pretense may lead the patient to feel depressed and alone; open awareness is marked with beneficial family dynamics, realistic thinking and goal setting and final planning.

Nurses can help the patient and the family members to achieve open awareness within an open and trusting environment in which the patient and family members are able to fully and openly express their fears and feelings.

SUPPORTING ADVANCE CARE PLANNING

Advance care planning typically consists of a durable power of attorney for health care, or health care surrogate, a living will, advance medical care directives and a patient-completed values history. Most often, the advance medical care directive consists of both the living will and the durable power of attorney for health care. Ideally, all of these decisions and documents should be done when the patient is competent and healthy so they can be well thought out and complete.

Durable Power of Attorney for Healthcare

A durable power of attorney for health care, also referred to as a healthcare proxy or healthcare surrogate, is a legally appointed person who will make decisions relating to healthcare when the patient is no longer competent and able to give legal consent.

Advance Medical Care Directives

Advance medical care directives, also referred to as living wills and advance directives, contain the wishes of the patient in terms of treatments and interventions that they do and do not want carried out when they are no longer able to competently provide consent. For example, a patient with cancer may choose to have tube feedings but no IVs in their advanced directive.

The most commonly seen components of advance directives include choices relating to life support measures, mechanical ventilation, intravenous solution administration and methods of artificial feeding, like tube feedings. Many patients at the end of life choose DNR (do not resuscitate), and they specifically state that they do not want mechanical ventilation, intravenous fluids and/or tube feedings.

These directives should be as specific and complete as possible. When an unanticipated event or treatment occurs that is not included in the advance directive, decisions are made by the durable power of attorney for healthcare in the best interests of the patient and their values.

Values Histories

Values histories further support the patient's beliefs and opinions in terms of healthcare decisions that were not documented in the person's living will, especially when the durable power of attorney for healthcare needs guidance. For example, has the patient expressed feelings about life without pain? Has the patient expressed beliefs about wanting to die with dignity? Although many healthcare patients do not have a values history, it is highly recommended.

DISASTER PREPAREDNESS

Respiratory therapists play an important role in internal and external disasters and emergency preparedness.

INTERNAL DISASTERS

Examples of internal disasters include fires, power losses, tornados, workplace violence, cyclones, hurricanes, and explosions. These situations are life endangering; there is little time to think and react.

FIRES

In order for fires to start it is necessary to have heat, air, and something to burn. If all three are not present, fire cannot start, so a way to prevent fires is to eliminate one of these three things. For example, a fire can be prevented when an open flame (heat) is not allowed near oxygen (gas that burns) in a room filled with air; fire can also be prevented when cigarette smoking (heat) is not permitted in patient rooms or in beds (something that burns.) Other things that can burn can be a solid, like paper and wood, a liquid, like grease, a gas such as kerosene fumes, and electricity.

Fire prevention includes facility-wide smoke detectors and fire sprinklers, as well as established policies and procedures relating to smoking, oxygen use, electrical safety and the use of other gases like nitrous oxide. Facilities also have established policies and procedures to deal with fires and other internal and external disasters should they occur. All members of the facility must be fully knowledgeable about these procedures because when a disaster occurs there is no time to read the manual. Immediate action is necessary.

You MUST act quickly if a fire starts. You must R-A-C-E.

- *Rescue* everyone in danger; get all patients and visitors out of danger by following the fire plan set up by the facility you work in.

- *Alarm* – the fire alarm MUST be pulled.

- *Confine* or contain the fire. Close all doors and windows; fire doors are supposed to automatically close to contain a fire in a small area and to prevent its spread to other areas of the facility.

- *Extinguish* the fire, only if it is safe to do so and there is no possibility that you can injure yourself or anyone else. Small fires can be put out with water when it is a solid, like paper, that is burning or a fire extinguisher. If the fire is too large to handle, get out and wait for professional firefighters or your facility's fire squadron.

When a fire occurs, you may be instructed to evacuate patients. The two methods of evacuation are vertical and horizontal. When you are instructed to do a vertical evacuation, you will move patients from one floor to another. For example, when a fire breaks out on the 4th floor, you will be instructed to move the patients to a lower level than the 4th floor because smoke and fire spreads upward. When you are instructed to horizontally evacuate patient, you will move the patients from one area of the floor to another area on the same floor as far away from the fire as possible.

All medical facilities must have emergency evacuation plans and they should be posted so that they can be referred to, and followed, in a rapid manner. Elevators are never used during a fire emergency. Elevators are reserved for fire fighters and other emergency personnel, and, elevators can lose electricity and trap people inside during a fire. The stairway is the only path of exit that can be used. For obvious reasons, many patients will need assistance during vertical evacuations.

If a fire is blocking a patient's exit from their room, the door should be shut to keep the fire out of the room and a towel or blanket should be placed at the bottom of the door to keep the smoke out of their room.

If a fire alarm sounds when you and/or your patient are in the room with the door closed, you must feel the door before opening it. A hot door means that the fire is just on the other side of the door so leave the door closed. Do not open it; instead, put a towel or blanket at the bottom of the door to keep the smoke out, and call for help.

Fire Extinguishers

All medical facilities must have fire extinguishers. There are several different types of fire extinguishers, which include:

- *Type A*: This extinguisher can only be used to put out fires on common solid things like paper, wood and cloth; they CANNOT be used on oil, grease or electrical fires.

- *Type B*: Type B fire extinguishers are used to put out fires on liquids and gases like gasoline, oil and grease. It can be used on kitchen grease and fat fires. It CANNOT be used on electrical fires.

- *Type C*: This extinguisher can is used to put out electrical fires.

- *Type AB*: Type AB fire extinguishers are a combination of a type A and type B fire extinguisher.

- *Type BC*: Similar to the type AB fire extinguisher which is a combination of types A and B fire extinguishers, type BC fire extinguishers are a combination of the types B and C fire extinguishers.

- *Type ABC*: This fire extinguisher is the best of all; it puts out all kinds and types of fires. It is highly recommended that these be in every healthcare facility and in the home. They can be bought at almost every home improvement store for very little cost.

It is required that all fire extinguishers be checked regularly to see that they are fully charged and ready to use in an emergency. To use a fire extinguisher, the P-A-S-S method is used, which is as follows:

- *Pull* the pin

- *Aim* at the base, or the bottom, of the fire or flame

- *Squeeze* the trigger while holding the extinguisher up straight and

- *Sweep,* or move the spray, from side to side to completely cover the fire

What To Do When a Patient's Clothes are on Fire

The rule for this disaster is to STOP, DROP AND ROLL. Tell the patient, or any other person, to STOP and DROP and NOT run. Running will add air to the fire and make it more serious. Tell them to lie down on the floor and to cover their face with their hands as you then roll them over and over again to smother the flames. You should also cover the person with a blanket or another item to put out the flames and smother the fire. Do NOT fan a fire with your hands. This, like running, will only make the fire worse.

Smoke

If a room fills with smoke, the rule is to GET LOW AND GO. Smoke will fill a room from the ceiling down. The patients and visitors MUST get to the floor and crawl. As mentioned earlier, the door should be felt for heat and, if it is safe to exit the room, everyone should cover their nose and mouth with a wet rag and crawl out of the area and out of danger.

TORNADOS AND SERIOUS HURRICANES

The following are steps that must be taken in case of a tornado:

- *Go to the lowest level of the building near the center of an interior room that has no windows, doors or outside walls. Do NOT open windows. Close them quickly if you can. These measures protect people from flying debris.*

- *Evacuate if you are told to do so. Close all interior doors.*

- *Keep curtains and blinds closed*

- *Cover your face and head with your arms and crouch down*

- *Cover your mouth with a handkerchief or clothing to keep dust out if you become trapped under fallen objects*

TERRORISM

Terrorism is described as the use of violence and force against people and property by non-state actors in the pursuit of political aims. There are several different types of terrorism, such as chemical, biological, nuclear and radiological weapons, all of which can lead to death and serious health problems.

If an act of terrorism occurs in your facility, you MUST follow the instructions given to you by the facility because responses to these acts vary greatly in terms of the type of act and the severity. For example, you may be simply advised to be aware of your surroundings and to stay in place while the police search for a bomb after a telephone threat has been received.

EXTERNAL DISASTERS

Examples of external disasters include massive flooding, a nuclear explosion or a major train/bus accident. The roles of healthcare professionals within a given organization vary, so it is important that you are familiar with your organization's policies, procedures and protocols relating to disasters.

TRIAGE PROCEDURES

All members must respond rapidly to external disasters that bring large numbers of victims with varying needs and little or no warning. In most cases, victims are transported to the hospital after they have been field-triaged. Color coded tags are often used to denote the severity of arriving victims:

Black Expectant	Pain medication only until expected death
Red Immediate	Life threatening injuries
Yellow Delayed	Non-life threatening injuries
Green Minimal	Minor injuries

EQUIPMENT AND SUPPLY MANAGEMENT

Supplies and equipment should not have to be checked and stocked during an emergency or another disaster. They should be inventoried and stocked on a regular and ongoing basis so that they are ready before the worst-case scenario materializes. After a massive external disaster, it is necessary to again inventory, restock and reorder supplies and equipment.

INTERACTING WITH THE INTERDISCIPLINARY TEAM

Patient care is very complex and positive outcomes can only be achieved when there is ongoing professional collaboration and cooperation among many members of the healthcare team, as well as financial experts within the facility. In addition to the benefits of collaboration in terms of patient care and outcomes, collaboration also enhances commitments, creative problem solving, consensus, and productivity.

For example, a respiratory therapist may collaboratively care for patients to facilitate access to wellness promotion in consultation and collaboration with a dietician (diet), patient educator (education relating to the components of wellness), a physical therapist (an exercise routine) and a social worker to determine the availability of community resources. Likewise, a respiratory therapist will collaborate with a pediatrician, social worker, patient educator and a utilization manager when a young mother must have access to healthcare services in order to prevent their children from becoming ill.

CRITICAL THINKING AND DECISION MAKING

The respiratory care process consists of assessment, planning, implementation, and evaluation. The assessment and evaluation phases entail the collection of objective, or empirical, data, and subjective data.

Subjective data is not measurable or observable and typically consists of the patient's own words. For example, a statement from the patient about their dyspnea is an example of subjective data. Objective data, on the other hand, is measurable and empirically observable and measurable. Vital signs and arterial blood gases, for example, are objective data. Evaluating and monitoring the patient's objective and subjective responses to respiratory care are done as part of the evaluation phase.

When the necessary data is available, this data is used; when sufficient data to evaluate and monitor the patient's response is not available, the respiratory therapist will collect it or recommend that it be collected.

Some of the subjective data that are collected to be evaluated and monitored in terms of the patient's responses to respiratory care include patient comments about their dyspnea, discomfort, and the efforts it takes to breathe.

Among other data, some of the objective data that are collected to evaluate and monitor the patient's responses to respiratory care include:

- *The results of a chest radiograph*

- *Arterial blood gases*

- *Arterialized capillary blood*

- *Pulmonary function test results*

Some of the subjective data that are collected to evaluate and monitor the patient's responses to respiratory care include patient comments about their dyspnea, discomfort, and the effort it takes to breathe.

CARE MODIFICATION

As discussed immediately above, the respiratory therapist recommends a wide variety of care modifications as based on the current status of the patient and they also independently modify care as based on their assessments within the scope of their practice.

EVALUATING EDUCATION AND PATIENT UNDERSTANDING

Health education is an important aspect of health promotion because it facilitates the individual's or group's ability to make knowledgeable decisions and motivates behavioral change by influencing values and beliefs.

THE DOMAINS OF LEARNING

There are three domains of learning that are the basis of all education, including patient and family education. These domains are:

- *The Cognitive Domain*

  This domain consists of both knowledge and understanding. An example of a cognitive domain patient outcome is, "The patient verbalized knowledge of all of their medications and side effects."

  The six levels of the cognitive domain from the most basic to the most complex are knowledge, comprehension, application, analysis, synthesis and evaluation. Some of the teaching/learning strategies for this domain include online/computer based learning, peer group discussions, reading material and a discussion or lecture.

- *The Psychomotor Domain*

  The psychomotor domain consists of "hands-on skills" like using an incentive spirometer accurately and using a blood glucose monitor correctly.

  The seven levels of this domain are perception, set, guided response, mechanism, complex overt response, adaptation and origination. Some of the teaching/learning strategies for this domain include demonstration, return demonstration and a video with a step-by-step demonstration of the psychomotor skill.

- *The Affective Domain*

The affective domain includes the development of attitudes, beliefs, values and opinions. An example of affective domain competency is developing a belief that exercise is a valuable part of wellness.

There are five levels, which are receiving, responding, valuing, organization and characterization by a value or a value complex. The teaching/learning strategies for this domain include role-playing and values clarification exercises. The affective domain is rarely used for patient teaching.

THE TEACHING PROCESS

Phase	Purpose	Components
Assessment	The purpose of assessment is to collect data about the learner(s) and their actual or potential learning needs. Within the community, the target group is identified and their learning needs are assessed. The assessment phase should include the identification of learning needs and the identification of influences that can impact on the	Assess the learner's: • current knowledge/skill • strengths/weaknesses • health beliefs • existing barriers to learning and behavior change • level of motivation • health problems • age-related/cultural characteristics • preferences/learning style • learning need The dimensions model helps assess and address the following factors: • biophysical • psychological • physical environment • sociocultural • behavioral

	learning process.	• health services

Planning	The purpose of planning is to analyze data to create learning goals/strategies, necessary content, and a teaching plan consistent with the learner's needs, preferences and characteristics, including cultural beliefs/practices, language/literacy, and health literacy level.	Planning consists of: • establishing priorities • determining and developing learning goals and objectives • selecting an appropriate teaching/learning strategy • selecting, organizing and developing content
Implementation	The purpose of implementation is to execute the teaching plan.	Implementation may involve a lecture or a video, for example.
Evaluation	The purpose of evaluation is to determine whether or not the individual or group has met the pre-established learning goals. Evaluation allows us to assess the teaching and learning processes and to determine its effects on the	Evaluation can be done by using a test or oral questioning (cognitive domain) or by asking the person to demonstrate a behavior or skill (psychomotor domain), depending on which domain of learning was addressed with the education.

	health of the learner.	

BARRIERS TO LEARNING

ILLITERACY OR POOR READING SKILLS

Sadly, many people in our nation are not able to read at all. Some may only be able to read and comprehend material at a low-grade level. It is sometimes recommended that patient education material be authored at or below 6th grade reading level to accommodate for these comprehension and literacy needs. Healthcare professionals must assess the patient's literacy level and provide learning materials that are appropriate to the patient in terms of their reading level so that the person is able to benefit from them.

LACK OF HEALTH LITERACY

Patients are considered "health literate" when they are able to understand information and use it to make appropriate health care decisions. Almost 50% of patients are NOT health literate.

Healthcare professionals must modify their communication and teaching to accommodate for this weakness and to ensure comprehension. For example, simple anatomy and physiology information relating to infection is preferred over complex, biochemical explanations that the patient cannot understand. Additionally, the use of medical jargon and terminology should be avoided.

LACK OF MOTIVATION OR READINESS

Patients will not learn unless they are motivated and ready to do so. Healthcare professionals can motivate learners by involving them in the entire teaching/learning process, by focusing the learning on solving immediate and pressing concerns, and by explaining the benefits of learning in terms of problem resolution, while maintaining an environment that is supportive of an open, honest and highly respectful learning environment.

Motivation to learn and motivation to change are assessed as part of the assessment phase of the teaching process.

DIFFERING LEARNING STYLES AND PREFERENCES

Individual learning styles and preferences should be accommodated for as often as possible. Some individuals are auditory or visual learners; some learn best by reading or by doing. Some like to read, or watch a video, or use a computer; others do not.

INCOMPATIBLE CULTURAL CONSIDERATIONS

Communication patterns, vocabulary, slang and/or terminology, are differences that can separate the members of a group or culture from those who are not members. Healthcare professionals must become culturally competent about the norms of others and also modify their terminology and behavior according to what is acceptable and understandable to the learner of a different culture.

AGE-SPECIFIC CHARACTERISTICS

Some examples of teaching modifications based on age are simple concrete and brief explanations for the toddler, simple and brief explanations for the pre-school child, the encouragement of questions and more detailed explanations for the school age child, and adult like teaching for the adolescent.

LANGUAGE BARRIERS

When there is a language barrier, communicating and teaching can be difficult. Several simple techniques can help overcome these barriers, such as speaking slowly, clarifying, re-clarifying, using pictures and diagrams, and eliciting the help of an interpreter.

INCORRECT HEALTH BELIEFS

Health beliefs can also be a barrier to learning and changes in behavior. Patients who place a high value on health, health promotion and wellness will be more motivated to learn.

INCOMPATIBLE RELIGIOUS AND SPIRITUAL ISSUES

Religious and spiritual beliefs can include the use of symbols, dreams, spiritual practices and beliefs, including those that are metaphysical in nature.

For example, maintaining health may involve the use of proper diet (physical facet), the support of others (psychological facet) and things like meditation, prayer and formalized religious practices (spiritual facet.)

Similarly, health protection can be facilitated with symbolic clothing and special spiritual foods (physical facet), the avoidance of people and things that can lead to disease (psychological facet), and the use of religious customs and amulets like the "Evil Eye" to ward off evil and harm (spiritual facet.)

Lastly, the restoration of health is enabled with alternative healing methods, such as massage, herbs, homeopathic remedies and special foods (physical facet), exorcism, the use of culturally traditional healers, like medicine men and *curanderos* (spiritual facet), relaxation techniques (psychological facet) and religious rituals or special prayers.

UNHEALTHY FAMILY DYNAMICS AND OTHER SOCIAL FORCES

Many patients have social support systems and family supports; however many lack these supports. For example, the patient may be widowed, single, geographically separated from family and friends, and/or may not have family or friends that support them and their need for education and behavior changes.

PSYCHOLOGICAL FACTORS

Healthcare professionals have to assess and accommodate for any actual or potential cognitive, sensory and psychological/emotional barriers to learning. For example, cognitive limitations can be overcome with slow, brief, simple and understandable explanations.

Psychological barriers can be minimized by establishing trust, reinforcing learning with positive feedback, and minimizing stress. Moderate stress is a motivator; extreme stress and pain prevent learning. For this reason, extreme stress and pain should be addressed before the educational activity.

COMPROMISED PHYSICAL CAPABILITIES AND PHYSICAL LIMITATIONS

Sensory barriers can be accommodated for with large print materials and Braille for the visually impaired, louder discussions with patients affected with a hearing loss, and the use of assistive devices like eyeglasses and hearing aids.

Functional limitations can also impede learning. For example, a patient who has lost fine motor coordination may not be able to draw up their own insulin without the help of some assistive devices. Healthcare professionals have to assess and accommodate for any actual or potential cognitive, sensory and psychological/emotional barriers to learning.

Cognitive limitations can be overcome with slow, brief, simple and understandable explanations. Sensory barriers can be accommodated for with large print materials and Braille for the visually impaired, louder discussions with patients affected with a hearing loss, and the use of assistive devices like magnifiers, eyeglasses and hearing aids. Psychological barriers can be minimized with establishing trust, reinforcing learning with positive feedback, and minimizing stress. Moderate stress is a motivator; extreme stress and pain prevent learning.

THE ASSESSMENT PHASE

The purpose of assessment is to determine the patient's learning needs, their level of motivation and readiness, personal, ethnical and cultural aspects, age specific characteristics and needs, barriers to learning including cognitive impairments, language, level of comprehension or reading level, and physical as well as psychological barriers to learning. Simply stated, a learning need equals what should be known, subtracting what is actually known. Educational needs can be expressed as "A lack of knowledge about...", and "A knowledge deficit related to...", for example.

Learning goals are statements regarding the expected behavior change that the teaching episode should facilitate. They are established during the planning phase of the patient and family education process, to guide the teaching progress and enable objective evaluation of outcomes and effectiveness. For example, a goal may be practicing safe sex. Learning objectives, or outcomes, reflect what the person will know, or do, during and after the teaching episode. These objectives or outcomes reflect the steps that the person must do, or know, in order to reach the ultimate goal.

Learning objectives must be:

- *Learner-oriented*
- *Specific*
- *Measurable and behavioral*
- *Consistent with the domain and level of knowledge*
- *Consistent with assessed need*

Appropriate LOs	Inappropriate LOs
Learner Oriented: The learner will be able to describe the components of proper hand washing.	Teacher-Oriented: The healthcare professional will instruct the patient about proper hand washing.
Specific: The learner will be able to list the steps of hand washing.	Non-Specific: The learner will be able discuss hand washing.

Measurable/ Behavioral: The learner will correctly demonstrate the procedure for proper hand washing.	Non Measurable & Non Behavioral: The learner will be able understand hand washing.
Consistent With Learning Domain: The learner will be able to properly demonstrate the hand washing procedure.	Inconsistent With Learning Domain: The learner will be able to describe the proper hand washing procedure.
Consistent With Level of Domain: Categorize the level of risk associated with multiple and complex risk factor relationships	Inconsistent With Level of Domain: List the degree of risk associated with multiple and complex risk factor relationships

Begin the learning objective with the statement "At the conclusion of the teaching, the learner will be able to..." The statement should start with a measurable verb consistent with the domain of learning and domain level, such as those below:

Cognitive Domain	Psychomotor Domain	Affective Domain
• **Define** • **Describe** • **Identify** • **Discuss** • **Summarize** • **Outline**	• Use • Perform • Demonstrate	• Can demonstrate a belief • Complies • Accepts • Values

THE PLANNING PHASE

Generally speaking, when planning, content and information should be sequenced from the known to the unknown, from the simple to the complex and from the least threatening to the most threatening.

For example, when the healthcare professional wants to teach about the chain of infection, the educator will sequence the content and information to move the patient from information about the basic ways that infections can be spread (simple and known) to the characteristics of a susceptible host (complex and unknown.) Additionally, when teaching the patient about changing a surgical dressing, the educator will allow the patient to practice dressing techniques on a medical model (less threatening) and then move the patient to change their own dressing (more threatening.)

The knowledge, skills and abilities will also be sequenced according to the levels of complexity for each of the domains of learning. Teaching strategies must be selected based on the domain of learning being taught. For example, lecture and discussion are appropriate strategies for the cognitive domain and demonstration, return demonstration and practice are appropriate strategies for the psychomotor domain. Content is also developed in order to ensure that it is current, accurate and appropriate to the learning need. Healthcare professionals must also be able to apply the principles of adult learning to patients and family members. Pedagogy is childhood learning; andragogy is adult learning. Unlike pedagogy, adult learning has immediate usefulness in terms of solving problems; it involves active learner involvement and participation; and the curriculum and content are based on the learner's needs and desires.

	Pedagogy	Andragogy
Curriculum	The state and the teacher develop and design the teaching, based on what they decide is important.	The learner, in collaboration with the diabetes educator, develops and designs the teaching, based on learner needs and characteristics, such as their preferred learning style.
Level of Input	The child is a somewhat passive learner. The learner has a low level of involvement in all the phases of the teaching process.	The adult is a highly active learner. The learner has a high level of involvement in all the phases of the teaching process.
Teaching Methods	Homework & Teacher Lecture	Active learner participation The adult learner has a large amount of knowledge and experiences to share with others and to relate to the learning activity.
Purpose of Learning	Childhood learning has little immediate application. This learning prepares the child for the future and their future needs.	Adult learning should have immediate application and usefulness. The learning aims to solve problems.

THE IMPLEMENTATION PHASE

In the implementation phase, the educator actually teaches the class using a variety of teaching strategies, also known as teaching methodologies. These must be consistent with the learning need, objectives, styles(s), and the domain and level of domain that needs addressed.

Cognitive Domain	Psychomotor Domain	Affective Domain
• Online Learning • Workshops • Lecture • Discussion • Videos • Reading Materials • Games • Posters or Pictures	• Live Demonstration • Video Demonstration • Step-by-Step Pictures • Simulations • Use of Medical Models	• Role Playing

Regardless of experience, many educators encounter problems with the planning and duration of a teaching session. To adequately plan for teaching/learning interaction, instructors should abide by the following principles:

For patients who learn best through psychomotor methods, short teaching sessions that demonstrate each step of the procedure or process are helpful. Allowing ample time between learning sessions enables the patient to practice alone without the added stress of another's prescence. This is particularly helpful when the learner has an impairment.

For patients who suffer from short-term memory loss as a result of natural aging processes or other factors, more time and greater repetition is beneficial for the patient or family member(s.) Those with short attention spans, such as children, the cognitively impaired and those with a serious illness or pain should be brief and modified, based on the individual's need.

As with the types of patients discussed above, most patients benefit from multiple short sessions over time. For example, if a patient needs to learn discharge instructions, a brief session about the medications the patient will take when discharged on day one and then another session the next day on beneficial community resources they can utilize will enable the patient to internalize information better.

When working with groups, particularly if they are mixed groups of varying knowledge or large groups, more time for a teacher session is needed than with homogenous or smaller groups.

THE EVALUATION PHASE

There are two types of evaluation in the teaching/learning process. They are referred to as formative and summative evaluation.

Formative evaluation is the continuous assessment of how effective the learning is during the timeframe in which the activity is implemented. Formative evaluation enables the teacher to modify the teaching plan if, during the course of learning, it is determined that the outcomes are not being achieved successfully.

If the formative evaluation is unsatisfactory, consider whether:

- *There are any learning barriers the plan did not assess or consider*

- *The time allocation is adequate*

- *The reading material is at the appropriate reading level of the patient*

- *The environment promotes learning*

- *The learner is committed to the learning objectives*

- *The learning objectives were realistic*

- *The teaching methodology is appropriate*

FACTORS IMPEDING LEARNING

Summative evaluation helps determines whether the education has achieved its established objectives.

If one or more learning objectives were not achieved, the education was ineffective, meaning the teacher must:

1) return to the assessment phase to validate the accuracy of assessed needs,

2) then return to the planning phase to determine if this phase is educationally sound, and

3) make necessary modifications to achieve desired outcomes during future re-teaching sessions.

It is important to note that learning is not always permanent. As a result, health care providers should periodically assess the patient to determine if the patient has retained the knowledge or skill. If the knowledge or skill has not been retained, learning reinforcement is needed.

Summative evaluation strategies that are suitable for each domain include:

Cognitive Domain	Psychomotor Domain	Affective Domain
• Oral Questioning • Written Tests	• Return Demonstration	• Changed Belief, Attitude or Value

LONG-TERM AND AGGREGATED EVALUATION

Some questions you can ask to perform a long-term summative, or aggregated evaluation include:

- *Has the learner(s) retained the knowledge over time?*

- *Did the patient contact the physician if they had a suspected adverse drug reaction to their antibiotic?*
- *Has the number of readmissions secondary to surgical wound infections decreased after individualized teaching about wound care and sterile dressing changes?*
- *Has the number of immunizations for pediatric patients increased?*
- *Has the education helped to decrease the lengths of stay for resistant pathogen affected patients?*
- *Has the education decreased postoperative pneumonia in the facility?*
- *Has the rate and frequency of unexpected returns to the emergency room or primary physician decreased?*
- *Have customer satisfaction scores increased?*

The answers to these questions should indicate a change in behavior, which is the purpose of education. This change in behavior needs to be measurable for individuals and groups.

If a patient teaching plan is successful, it is recommended that the entire facility work to adopt it as the standard to ensure no variation in process and to ensurethat successful outcomes are maintained and predictable.

DISCHARGE TEACHING

Patients who are discharged to the home must receive education and training according to their assessed learning needs. Some of this teaching includes the knowledge, skills and abilities to:

- *Perform tracheostomy care*
- *Monitor the patient's status*
- *Perform CPR*
- *Use ordered equipment*
- *Administer and manage medications*

Perform Tracheostomy Care

Performing tracheostomy care is a psychomotor skill that should be taught with a demonstration. After demonstration and practice, the learner, typically the parent, should be able to perform correct tracheostomy care.

Monitor the Patient's Status

The learner will need education relating to cognitive aspects as well as some psychomotor aspects. For example, the learner should be able to observe the signs and symptoms of respiratory distress, which is a cognitive skill, and also be able to take and record the vital signs, which is a psychomotor skill.

Perform CPR

It is recommended that the parents of children with chronic lung disorders take the American Heart Association's course on pediatric CPR.

Use Ordered Equipment

The proper use of ordered equipment and troubleshooting should be taught before discharge to the home.

Administer and Manage Medications

Discharge teaching includes information about all the medications that the infant or child will be taking in the home. Some of the components of this teaching include the medication:

- *Actions*
- *Dosage*
- *Route*

- *Frequency*
- *Side effects*
- *Adverse actions*

COMMON ISSUES REQUIRING NPS-SPECIFIC EDUCATION

SURFACTANT

Surfactant, which is composed of lecithin and sphingomyelin, lowers the alveolar surface tension so the alveoli are stabilized and a certain amount of air remains in the alveoli after expiration during extrauterine life. The risk factors associated with a surfactant deficiency include premature neonates without full lung development and patients affected with cystic fibrosis, asthma, bronchitis, pneumonia, aspiration, pulmonary hemorrhage, respiratory syncytial infection, sepsis, smoke inhalation, trauma, shock and trauma like a near drowning.

The physiological signs and symptoms of a surfactant deficiency include atelectasis, a decreased functional residual capacity, tachypnea, cyanosis, poor perfusion, apnea, nasal flaring, diminished breath sounds, retractions, grunting and other signs of respiratory distress.

Laboratory values will show that the patient is affected with metabolic acidosis, a decrease Po_2 and increased carbon dioxide. Radiographic imaging may show atelectasis and diffuse reticular granular patterns.

The goal of treatment for a surfactant deficiency secondary to another physical disorder is the treatment of the underlying disorder and supportive respiratory care as indicated.

Some research indicates that the administration of prophylactic surfactant for low weight and preterm neonates within moments after delivery can prevent pneumothorax, pulmonary interstitial emphysema and mortality. When prophylaxis is not given, treatment with surfactant is indicated with the onset of symptoms in addition to intubation and respiratory support.

MECONIUM ASPIRATION

Fetal stress, such as placental insufficiency or hypoxia secondary to an umbilical cord compression, leads to meconium aspiration. Neonates can also aspirate vernix caseosa, amniotic fluid, as well as maternal or fetal blood.

Post term infants delivered with low amounts of amniotic fluid are at greatest risk because the meconium is less dilute and more concentrated.

The signs and symptoms include rales, rhonchi, tachypnea, cyanosis, desaturation and respiratory distress as the result of mechanical bronchial obstruction and inflammatory pneumonitis.

The diagnosis is made in the presence of respiratory distress, meconium stained amniotic fluid and is confirmed with a chest x-ray, which can show hyperinflation, areas of atelectasis and a flattening of the neonate's diaphragm.

Meconium aspiration is a life threatening emergency. Treatment includes immediate suctioning after birth with DeLee suctioning, supplemental oxygen, antibiotics and respiratory support as needed. In some cases, endotracheal intubation and mechanical ventilation may be indicated.

Depressed respirations, a pulse of less than 100 beats/min and poor muscle tone signal the urgency of endotracheal intubation with a 3.5 to 4.0-mm endotracheal tube and continuous positive airway pressure followed by mechanical ventilation. Surfactant, inhaled nitric oxide from 5 to 20 ppm and extracorporeal membrane oxygenation are often administered to mechanically ventilated neonates.

Infants affected with meconium aspiration at the time of birth are at risk for the development of asthma as they grow older.

ASPIRATION PNEUMONIA

Aspiration pneumonia occurs when meconium, food, saliva, liquids, or vomit is breathed into the lungs or airways leading to the lungs. This disease can lead to lung abscesses, shock, septicemia and respiratory failure. The risk factors associated with aspiration pneumonia include decreased levels of consciousness, a poor gag reflex and prematurity.

The signs and symptoms include those associated with an airway obstruction such as compromised respiratory status, hypoxia, cyanosis, wheezing, tachycardia, retraction and possible respiratory failure.

The diagnosis is made based on the signs and symptoms, chest x-ray and other imaging studies, bronchoscopy and the analysis of arterial blood gases.

Depending on the severity, the patient may require antibiotics, oxygen supplementation, suctioning and mechanical ventilation. Additionally, the underlying disorder should also be corrected and treated whenever possible.

PERSISTENT PULMONARY HYPERTENSION OF THE NEWBORN (PPHN)

This life-threatening disorder diverts blood flow from the lungs and seriously compromises the neonate's level of oxygenation. The symptoms typically appear 72 hours after birth and it can affect all neonates including full term babies. The risk factors associated with PPHN include meconium aspiration, infection, hypothermia and congenital lung and heart diseases.

The signs and symptoms include grunting upon exhalation, tachypnea, retractions, cyanosis, pallor, hypoxemia, scant urinary output and edema.

Supplemental oxygen with an oxygen hood, continuous positive air pressure (CPAP), continuous mechanical ventilation, high frequency ventilation, sedation, antibiotics as indicated, surfactant administration and extracorporeal membrane oxygenation are some of the treatment alternatives that are used as based on the severity of this disorder.

LUNG DISEASE OF PREMATURITY

Lung disease of prematurity is also referred to as bronchopulmonary dysplasia (BPD.) The current definition of bronchopulmonary dysplasia applies to infants who meet these criteria:

- *Gestational age < 32 weeks*
- *Supplemental oxygen need for < 28 days*
- *Oxygen dependency at 36 weeks*

The goal of treatment is to establish and maintain adequate gas exchange and oxygenation while decreasing the risk for infection. Some of the treatment options include supplemental oxygen therapy, ventilation, anti-inflammatory medications, the prevention of aspiration and the prompt treatment of any complications such as pulmonary hypertension.

BRONCHIOLITIS

Bronchiolitis is an acute viral infection that affects the lower respiratory tract. Most cases are caused by RSV; however, this infection can also occur as the result of measles, influenza A and B, parainfluenza 1 and 2, and adenovirus.

This infection descends downward from the upper respiratory tract to the bronchioles and the small bronchi; the resulting edema and inflammatory secretions can lead to partial and complete airway obstructions, alveolar air trapping and even atelectasis which can worsen with high oxygen concentrations. Pediatric patients less than 24 months of age are at greatest risk and the highest incidence occurs among infants less than 6 months of age.

Among the signs and symptoms are wheezing, crackles, prolonged expiration, tachypnea, retractions, apneic spells, circumoral pallor and cyanosis, fever and exhaustion.

The prognosis is good with supportive treatment, however, the cough may persist for up to one month. Some supportive measures include oxygen supplementation and intravenous fluid and electrolyte replacements as needed.

CONGENITAL HEART DISEASES

Congenital heart disease is the leading cause of infant and neonatal mortality and the most commonly occurring congenital anomaly.

The risk factors that contribute to the development of congenital heart disease are paternal age, maternal diseases and disorders such as rubella, systemic lupus erythematous and diabetes as well as maternal intake of teratogenic substances like isotretinoin, lithium and anticonvulsants.

Some of the genetic chromosomal abnormalities associated with congenital heart disease include monosomy X, also referred to as Turner syndrome, trisomy 21, trisomy 18 and trisomy 13; genetic deletions and mutations such as DiGeorge syndrome and Williams-Beuren syndrome, as well as single-gene defects such as Marfan syndrome, Holt-Oram syndrome and Noonan syndrome also contribute to the risk of congenital heart disorders.

These cardiac disorders are broadly classified as cyanotic and acyanotic and they can vary along a continuum with few if any symptoms to severe signs and symptoms, including cardiac arrest, collapse and in some cases, death:

- *Tetralogy of Fallot*
- *Pulmonary atresia*
- *Persistent truncus arteriosus*
- *Transposition of the great arteries*
- *Tricuspid atresia*
- *Total anomalous pulmonary venous return*

- *The acyanotic congenital heart disorders are:*
- *Ventricular septal defect*
- *Atrial septal defect*
- *Patent ductus arteriosus*
- *Atrioventricular septal defect*
- *Pulmonic stenosis*
- *Aortic stenosis*
- *Aortic coarctation*

- *Hypoplastic   left heart   syndrome Left-to-right shunt*

Tetralogy of Fallot

Of all of these cardiac defects, the Tetralogy of Fallot is the most serious. This cyanotic congenital heart disorder is a defect that has four abnormal structural and physiological defects:

- *An overriding aorta*
- *Ventricular septal defect*
- *Pulmonary stenosis*
- *Right ventricular hypertrophy*

The chest x-ray shows a classic boot shape and in many cases, the aortic arch is on the right side, rather than the left side. Neonates with pronounced pulmonary stenosis have right to left shunting, a possible arterial oxygen saturation of 60% and severe cyanosis shortly after birth when the ductus arteriosus closes; those with less severe cases have left to right shunting.

The ventricular septal defect causes equal pressures in both ventricles and the blood flow to the pulmonary vessels and the systemic vessels vary according to the systemic vascular resistance and the degree of pulmonary stenosis. The pulmonary output and hemodynamics change with these variations and this leads to "tet" spells, particularly among infants who are 2 to 4 months of age. These spells consist of:

- *Increasing cyanosis*
- *Exaggerated deep breathing or hyperpnea*
- *Crying and irritability*
- *A lower heart murmur intensity*

The treatment of "tet" spells consist of holding the infant in a knee-to-chest position to decrease venous blood return, the administration of morphine sulfate to lower the respiratory rate and to dilation of the pulmonary artery, the administration of supplemental oxygen, the provision of sodium bicarbonate to resolve the acidosis and pulmonary artery constriction, the administration of vasoconstrictors to increase the systemic vascular resistance and propranolol to decrease pulmonary artery spasms.

Some severely affected neonates need immediate surgery to correct the defect; others can be treated with an immediate dose to prostaglandin E1 to maintain a patent ductus arteriosus and to maintain good pulmonary blood flow by lowering the peripheral vascular resistance.

In addition to corrective surgery and prostaglandin E1, other treatments include suctioning, oxygen administration, intubation and ventilation. The surgical procedure, done with a cardiopulmonary bypass, entails closing the ventricular septal defect, widening of the right ventricular outflow tract and reconstruction or patching of the stenosed pulmonary artery. A Blalock-Taussig shunt to the pulmonary artery from the subclavian artery is also done when the infant is adversely affected with severe obstruction and stenosis.

The most commonly occurring complication of this surgery is junctional atrial tachycardia, a cardiac arrhythmia.

TOTAL ANOMALOUS PULMONARY VENOUS RETURN

Total anomalous pulmonary venous return is characterized by the draining of the pulmonary veins indirectly or directly into the right atrium because there are none of these veins in the left atrium. The end result of this abnormal drainage is the mixing of systemic and pulmonary blood, increased pressure in the right side of the heart and anomalies that are classified as:

- Cardiac: The pulmonary vein empties into the coronary sinus.

- Supracardiac: The pulmonary vein empties into the superior vena cava

- Infracardiac: The pulmonary vein empties into the inferior vena cava, the ductus venosus, the portal vein or the hepatic vein

- Mixed: a combination of the above

Post-surgical correction care includes intubation, mechanical ventilation, and PEEP to manage pulmonary edema.

ATRIAL SEPTAL DEFECT

Atrial septal defects affect the upper and lower section of the septum which separates the right and the left atria. Atrial septal defects include immature and undeveloped endocardial cushion, a defect in the septum itself and an incompetent foramen ovale which leads to regurgitation between the right and left atria. There is an increase in pulmonary flow and flow is shunted from the left to the right through the atrial septal defect. Although this defect can lead to congestive heart failure and right ventricular hypertrophy, most children may be not be symptomatic until school age.

Surgical repair can include a relatively simple cardiopulmonary bypass or a patch which closes the septum. Post-surgical management may include mechanical ventilation but always includes monitoring of pulse oximetry and blood gases, which should be normal after repair.

VENTRICULAR SEPTAL DEFECT

Similar to an atrial septal defect, a ventricular septal defect is an abnormal opening between the left and right ventricles. These defects can range from very small to so large that the septum is almost absent altogether. The blood typically shunts from the left to the right because the systemic vascular resistance is greater than the pulmonary vascular resistance and it occurs during ventricular systole. On some occasions, the left to right shunt reverses to a right to left shunt when the pulmonary pressure exceeds that of the systemic circulation. This phenomena of reversal is referred to as Eisenmenger syndrome.

When this septal defect does not close in a couple of years and the child is symptomatic, furosemide and digoxin may be indicated. Patients with ongoing pulmonary infections, pulmonary hypertension, poor physical growth and impaired Pao2 and Sao2 typically require surgical correction. Surgical palliation, rather than treatment, can be done with pulmonary banding that entails placing a Teflon strip around the pulmonary artery to decrease the extent of the left right shunting. This procedure facilitates the child's physical growth and allows the patient to stabilize before a total repair with a cardiopulmonary bypass is done with a patch, similar to that which is used for the repair of an atrial septal defect.

PATENT DUCTUS ARTERIOSUS

Patent ductus arteriosus, which most often occurs with prematurity, is the failure of the ductus arteriosus to close immediately after birth as an adaptation to extrauterine life when chemical, blood gases and hormones change. This disorder often presents among infants who have respiratory distress syndrome and/or are premature.

The blood flow moves from left to right from the aorta into the pulmonary artery as a result of this disorder. The difference between pre-ductal and post-ductal blood, as obtained with a temporal artery or right radial and umbilical artery, respectively, of more than 15mm Hg in addition to noninvasive pulse oximetry readings differences of more than 5% when the right hand (pre-ductal) and the left hand or lower extremities (post-ductal) are compared indicate the presence of patent ductus arteriosus. This condition leads to heart failure, pulmonary hypertension, impaired gas exchange and diminished lung mechanics.

The diagnosis is made with echocardiography and the treatments include maintaining the hemoglobin at the highest possible normal value, maintaining euvolemia and indomethacin with a single dose of 0.2 mg/kg during the first day of life followed with additional doses thereafter. Also, the addition of PEEP in ventilated neonates can decrease the left to right shunting and increasing the systemic blood flow.

Surgical repair to close the ductus arteriosus is most often done before the tenth day of life when indomethacin is not effective. Although some infants need ventilator support after surgery, most have adequate pulse oximetry and arterial blood gas values.

ATRIOVENTRICULAR SEPTAL DEFECT

An atrioventricular septal defect can be complete, transitional or partial. The complete form often occurs with Down syndrome although, at times, it is also coupled with asplenia or polysplenia syndrome.

Complete atrioventricular defects include a ventricular septal defect, a large atrial septal defect, a regurgitating AV valve left to right shunting and heart failure typically occurs by the 4th to 6th week of life. These anatomical abnormities lead to left-to-right shunting at both the ventricular and atrial levels and enlargements of all of the four chambers of the heart. Partial atrioventricular defects include an atrial septal defect, right heart enlargement, an AV valve deformity, but no ventricular shunting or ventricular septal defect. Transitional atrioventricular defects are characterized by an atrial septa defect, a ventral septal defect and mitral regurgitation.

Depending on the type and severity, other signs and symptoms are dyspnea, particularly when feeding the infant, impaired growth, tachypnea, heart murmurs, tachycardia, hepatomegaly, a loud 2nd heart sound, splitting of S2, a systolic murmur and/or a diastolic murmur.

The treatment includes surgical repair before 6 months of age when the infant is symptomatic and, when indicated, the treatment of any heart failure with medications such as digoxin, ACE inhibitors and diuretics. Asymptomatic patients with a partial defect can have delayed surgery until the infant is from 1 to 2 years.

PULMONIC STENOSIS

Pulmonic stenosis is a stricture obstructing the pulmonary outflow and blood flow from the right ventricle to the pulmonary artery during systole. Some cases are congenital and not discovered until the patient has reached adulthood, however, many children are symptomatic and in need of treatment. This stenosis can be just below the valve (infundibula stenosis) or in the valve itself.

This cardiac disorder often accompanies Tetralogy of Fallot. Some of the risk factors include Noonan syndrome which is similar to Turner syndrome except it is not a chromosomal defect and carcinoid syndrome.

Although many children may be symptomatic until later years, some of the signs and symptoms associated with pulmonic stenosis include an ejection cardiac murmur, syncope, angina, dyspnea, distended jugular veins, a right ventricular precordial heave and a left parasternal systolic thrill at the second intercostal space. The 1st heart sound is normal; the splitting of the 2nd heart sound is prolonged.

The diagnosis is made with a Doppler echocardiography, after which this disorder is graded as listed below:

- Mild: The peak gradient is < 36 mm Hg

- Moderate: The peak gradient is between 36 and 64 mm Hg

- Severe: The peak gradient is > 64 mm Hg

The ECG may or may not indicate a right bundle branch block and/or hypertrophy. Cardiac catheterization is indicated when the patient is affected with both infundibula and valvular pulmonic stenosis.

Some of the treatments can include balloon valvuloplasty or percutaneous valve replacement, preferably with a prosthetic rather than a mechanic al heart valve to reduce the risk of thrombosis.

AORTIC STENOSIS

Left ventricular outflow obstructions, such aortic stenosis, coarctation of the aorta, hypoplastic aortic arc and interrupted aortic arch, hamper the ejection of blood from the left ventricle. Valvular aortic stenosis can occur above the aortic valve, at the level of the aortic valve and below the aortic valve which are referred to as supravalvular stenosis, valvular stenosis and subvalvular stenosis, respectively.

Some of the signs and symptoms include myocardial hypertrophy, ventricular over distension, and congestive heart failure. When left arterial pressures are high, it can lead to the movement of blood through the foramen ovale from left to right. Some of the symptoms that occur include syncope, chest pain, and a systolic pressure gradient less than 50 mm Hg.

Neonates who are symptomatic during the first month of life and those with heart failure are the most serious and with significantly low cardiac output, and, as such, need immediate surgery and ventilator support. Surgical repair includes artificial valve replacement, the Ross procedure which is a pulmonary valve autograph, widening of the stenosis using a patch, or aortic valvuloplasty.

Pre-surgical management includes the administration of prostaglandin E1 with a dosage of 0.05 to 0.1 ug/kg/min to decrease ductal constriction.

COARCTATION OF THE AORTA

Coarctation of the aorta narrows the lumen of the aortic arch. It typically occurs near the ductus arteriosus and it leads to decreased flow distal to the obstruction, increased workload and increased left ventricular pressure.

The two broad classifications of coarctation of the aorta are pre-ductal and post-ductal. Pre-ductal coarctations are more serious than post-ductal coarctations and they are frequently coupled with other cardiac abnormalities such as ventricular septal defects and aortic stenosis.

Some of the signs and symptoms include cardiomegaly, pulmonary vascular congestion, tachypnea, dyspnea, irritability and upper limb hypertension; therefore, the upper and lower limb blood pressures should be taken and compared for any differences.

Again, preoperative prostaglandin E1 is given to decrease ductal constriction in addition to diuretics and inotropic medications for cardiac failure. A variety of surgical procedures, including a patch, a tubular graft bypass and an end to end anastomosis after the coarctation has been excised. Post-surgically, the lower body blood pressure and perfusion may still be less than the upper extremity; however, it is generally thought that a difference of less than 20 mm Hg and adequate lower body perfusion indicates resolution.

HYPOPLASTIC LEFT HEART SYNDROME

This syndrome includes a number of different anomalies that affect the left side of the heart from the mitral valve to the arch of the aorta. Along the continuum, the patient can be affected with stenosis and atresia of the mitral or aortic valves in addition to hypoplasia of the aortic arch and the accenting aorta. This syndrome is characterized by minimal or no output from the left atrium. Shunting can be left to right or right to left depending on the pulmonary and systemic resistance.

The chest x-ray will show it as a globular shape as the result of heart enlargement and pulmonary edema.

Preoperative prostaglandin E1 is given to prevent hypo-perfusion of the systemic and coronary circulation and to also prevent pulmonary over-circulation. These concerns can be treated with the administration of sub-ambient oxygen with a FIO2 of 0.17 to 0.21 to maintain oxygen saturation of 70 to 80% and hyperbaric therapy. The goal of hyperbaric therapy is to indirectly increase pulmonary vascular resistance by elevating the PaCO2 to create respiratory acidosis within a pH range of 7.15 to 7.30. Additionally, mechanical ventilation can be used to increase dead space and the addition of CO2 and PaCO2 reductions in the minute ventilation also helps. Unlike sub-ambient oxygen administration, hyperbaric therapy can only be used for patients who are intubated, paralyzed and/or heavily sedated patients so the inspired gas concentrations and the minute ventilation can be scrupulously monitored and controlled.

Surgical interventions are based on the patient and their pulmonary blood and systemic blood pressure balances. In essence, the type of surgery is based on the ratio of pulmonary to cardiac blood flow, or Qp/Qs, and oxygenation measurements. The three phases of surgery in sequential order are:

1. *The Norwood procedure*   3. *The Fontan procedure*

2. *The Glenn procedure*

SHOCK

Simply stated, shock is a condition where body tissue is not sufficiently perfused; the oxygen demands exceed the amount of oxygen available to the body. The four stages of shock are:

1. *Initial Stage*

   Hypoxia occurs as the result of hypo-perfusion. Lactic acid rises during this stage because of the oxygen deprivation.

2. *Compensatory Stage*

   The body attempts to reverse the condition with compensatory physiological mechanisms. Hyperventilation attempts to blow off the increasing carbon dioxide and raise the blood pH. Epinephrine and norepinephrine are released into the body by the arterial baroreceptors. The epinephrine causes the heart rate to increase and the norepinephrine increases the heart rate and it also leads to vasoconstriction. Anti-diuretic hormone (ADH) is also released to save the kidneys with vasopressin.

3. *Progressive Stage*

Compensatory mechanisms begin to fail. Sodium ions build up, potassium ions leak out, metabolic acidosis increases, blood remains in the capillaries, histamine is released, fluid and proteins leak into surrounding tissues, the blood thickens and vital bodily organs are severely threatened.

4. *Refractory Stage or Final Stage*

Once this stage has occurred shock can no longer be reversed; death is imminent.

Types of Shock

The types of shock include:

- *Cardiogenic shock*
- *Anaphylactic shock*
- *Septic shock*

- *Neurogenic shock*
- *Hypovolemic shock*
- *Obstructive shock*

Cardiogenic Shock

This form of shock occurs when the ventricles of the heart are not functioning properly; this malfunction leads to inadequate circulation and reduced cardiac output. The most common cause of cardiogenic shock is myocardial muscle damage secondary to a serious myocardial infarction. Some of the other causes are heart failure, cardiac valve problems, dysrhythmias, cardiomyopathy and myocarditis.

Peripheral vasoconstriction (which limits blood flow to vital organs like the heart and the brain,) hypotension, tachycardia, oliguria and lethargy are some of the signs and symptoms associated with cardiogenic shock.

Anaphylactic Shock

Anaphylactic shock, like septic and neurogenic shock, are broadly classified as forms of distributive shock. All forms of distributive shock occur when there is a loss of tone in venules and arterioles. This type of distributive shock occurs when the body's immune system over reacts with systemic circulatory relaxation. Anaphylactic shock most often occurs as the result of an allergic response to a medication, such as penicillin.

The signs and symptoms include massive relaxation of the blood vessels, decreased cardiac output, histamine release, a drop in blood pressure, pooling of venous blood, laryngeal edema, a rash, and a rapid bounding heartbeat.

If the cause of the anaphylaxis a medication, it must be immediately discontinued. For example, if the cause is an intravenous antibiotic, the IV must be immediately discontinued; if the cause is an oral medication, this is also discontinued. Adrenaline or noradrenaline are then given to reduce laryngeal edema, to constrict the vasculature and to reverse the shock.

Neurogenic Shock

Neurogenic shock results when the sympathetic nervous system shuts down. It is most often associated with blocked spinal nerve functioning secondary to a spinal cord injury or during the administration of a spinal anesthetic. The arterioles and venules are relaxed. Bradycardia, hypotension, syncope and fainting can occur.

The treatment aims to remove and correct the underlying cause. Intravenous sympathetic stimulation medications like as atropine are administered.

Septic Shock

Septic shock is a systemic, multisystem response to a serious infection; it is associated with a high incidence of morbidity and mortality. Some of the risk factors for septic shock include a surgical or invasive procedure infection, immunocompromise, leukemia, and lymphoma.

The most common pathogens are gram positive bacteria, like staphylococcus aureus and streptococcus pneumoniae, gram negative bacteria, such as Escherichia coli and pseudomonas aeruginosa, and other microorganisms such as a virus, fungus or parasites.

Some of the ways that infections, bacteremia, sepsis and septic shock can be prevented are to minimize the use of invasive procedures and treatments to the greatest extent possible. All invasive procedures, like surgery, endoscopy, and all invasive treatments, like central lines, intravenous lines, and urinary catheters place patients at risk for an infection.

Massive vasodilation, cardiac depression, the formation of micro-emboli, and the abnormal distribution of intravascular fluid occur.

Early signs and symptoms include hypotension, flushed, warm skin, a widened pulse pressure, tachycardia, hyperventilation, metabolic acidosis, respiratory alkalosis, adventitious breath sounds like crackles, hypoxia, pulmonary edema, confusion and lethargy; late signs include highly serious decreases in cardiac output, peripheral vasoconstriction, and life threatening hypoxia that affects virtually all bodily systems.

Signs and symptoms of infection, such as a fever and an elevated white blood cell count, accompanied with hypotension, indicate the presence of septic shock. Hypotension accompanied by a bounding pulse is often the key clinical manifestation of sepsis.

Fluids are administered to restore fluid that has left the vascular spaces and to correct for the peripheral vasodilation. Other treatments can include mechanical ventilation, oxygen supplementation, possible dialysis, and medications including antibiotics for the infection, vasopressors such as noradrenaline medications to increase the blood pressure and ongoing hemodynamic monitoring.

Hypovolemic Shock

The stages of hypovolemic shock range from 1 to 4; stage 1 has minimal signs and symptoms and little blood loss; and stage 4 is characterized by severe clinical signs and symptoms and large blood losses greater than 40% of the patient's total circulating volume.

Hypovolemic shock is the most common type of shock. Primary, hypovolemic shock results from hemorrhage or the loss of fluid from the body's circulatory system. Patients at risk of this type of shock are those who suffer from burns, extreme dehydration, diabetic ketoacidosis, diabetes insipidus and those who have been exposed to environmental hazards.

The signs and symptoms that a patient may experience as a result of hypovolemic shock include pale skin, oral dryness, poor skin turgor and excessive thirst, which is a sign of dehydration being present, and due to the diminished circulating hemoglobin, tachypnea can occur.

The signs and symptoms vary according to the stage of the hypovolemic shock.

- Initial Stage: Hypoxia occurs as the result of hypo-perfusion.

- Compensatory Stage: Compensatory mechanisms such as hyperventilation (to raise PH and decrease carbon dioxide levels), decreased cardiac output (vasodilation), tachycardia (norepinephrine and epinephrine release), and diminished urinary output (anti-diuretic hormone release to protect the kidneys with vasopressin)

- Progressive Stage: Metabolic acidosis, increased blood viscosity with accompanying impaired microcirculation which severely compromises the perfusion of all vital organs (multisystem failure)

- Refractory or Irreversible Stage: Vital organs fail; death is imminent.

Ongoing assessments and the immediate correction of the cause (bleeding, dehydration) and the replacement of blood and fluid volume are necessary to preserve life. Hypovolemic shock is a life threatening event. Multiple intravenous catheters are placed and fluids like Lactated Ringers are administered at a rapid rate as well as blood, blood components and plasma expanders, as indicated.

Obstructive Shock

Obstructive shock occurs when there is an obstruction of the flow of blood outside of the heart into a major vessel, such as occurs when an embolus enters a major vessel. Obstructive shock, unlike other forms of shock, can affect relatively healthy people without any traumatic injury.

Like other forms of shock, the protective, compensatory baroreceptor reflexes protect the body's most essential organs at the expense of other bodily organs.

The signs and symptoms of obstructive shock include oliguria hypotension, tachycardia, and cyanosis.

The goal of treatment is to identify and correct the underlying cause such as a tension pneumothorax, aortic stenosis, cardiac tamponade or pulmonary embolism.

CARDIAC TAMPONADE

This life threatening emergency occurs when the pericardial sac rapidly collects fluid. This collection of fluid interferes with ventricular filling and pumping, and compression of the heart.

Signs and symptoms of cardiac tamponade include low urine output, tachycardia, mottled, cool skin, hypotension, a narrowed pulse pressure, weak peripheral pulses, muffled heart sounds, decreased level of consciousness, jugular vein distention and high central venous pressure.

This medical emergency requires hospitalization. Fluid in the pericardial sac is drained with a pericardicentesis. There are occasions when a portion or the pericardial sac is actually removed in order to relieve pressure on the patient's heart. Oxygen, intravenous fluids and medications are used to increase the patient's blood pressure and the underlying cause is corrected immediately after the patient is stabilized.

CYSTIC FIBROSIS

Cystic fibrosis is an inherited life threatening disease that results in severe damage to the lungs and digestive system. It is most commonly seen in white people of Northern European ancestry, but is also seen among Hispanics, African-Americans and in some Native Americans. It is rarely found among people who are Asian or Middle-Eastern.

Signs and symptoms can vary. A higher than normal level of salt in sweat is found in those with cystic fibrosis, and the other symptoms associated with cystic fibrosis affect the respiratory system and the digestive system. The thick and sticky mucous associated with cystic fibrosis affects the respiratory system with symptoms such as wheezing, breathlessness, decreased ability to exercise, inflamed nasal passages or a stuffy nose, and a persistent cough that produces thick sputum and mucus.

The thick mucus can also block the tubes that carry digestive enzymes from the pancreas to the small intestine. The intestines are unable to fully absorb the nutrients from the food without these essential digestive enzymes. This leads to nutritional and digestive impairments such as severe constipation, intestinal blockage, meconium ileus, poor growth and weight gain, and foul-smelling, greasy stools. Rectal prolapse can result from frequent straining associated with passing stools.

There is no cure for cystic fibrosis, so the aims of treatment are to prevent and control lung infections, loosen and remove mucus from the lungs, prevent and treat intestinal blockages, and to provide adequate nutrition.

Medications used for treatment include antibiotics, mucus thinning drugs, bronchodilators, and oral pancreatic enzymes. In addition to chest physical therapy to make it easier to cough up mucus, mechanical devices, such as chest clapper, inflatable vest, and breathing devices can be used.

Other treatment options include pulmonary rehabilitation, and surgical and other procedures, such as lung transplant, bowel surgery, feeding tube, endoscopy and lavage, oxygen therapy, and nasal polyp removal.

TRACHEOMALACIA

Tracheomalacia is the softening of the tracheal airway, narrowing of the airway or airway collapse. This disorder results from abnormal, defective cartilaginous support. The three types are:

I.   Congenital origin. Polychondritis and esophageal atresia are examples.

II. Acquired extrinsic compression. Cystic hygromas, tumors and vascular rings are some causes.

III. Acquired as the result of some inflammation and/or irritation such as gastroesophageal reflux disease and intubation.

The signs and symptoms include wheezing and stridor upon expiration.

This disorder can be self-resolving when the airway and its structure mature. In the interim, conservative treatment and support are indicated. More severe cases may lead to mortality as the result of respiratory complications such as desaturation, a failure to thrive, apnea, cyanosis and respiratory arrest as a result of V/Q mismatch. Aggressive treatment with bethanechol, tracheal stents, ipratropium bromide, CPAP, aortopexy and tracheostomy are indicated in severe cases.

SEIZURES

Seizures occur due to abnormal electrical activity in the brain. An epileptic seizure disorder, more commonly known as epilepsy, is a disorder in which a person has two or more unprovoked seizures. This brain disorder's cause is often unknown. Symptomatic epilepsy can be caused by strokes, tumors or malformations.

Seizures that are caused by temporary disorders or stressors are called non-epileptic seizures. Some of the causes are things like severe hypoglycemia, CNS infections, drug use or withdrawal, cardiovascular disorders and metabolic disorders. Seizures that occur due to a known cause, such as a stroke or brain tumor, are known as symptomatic seizures. These types of seizures are common mostly among the neonatal and elderly age groups

The two classifications of seizures are generalized seizures and partial seizures. Generalized seizures impair motor function throughout the seizure and the patient will usually become unconscious. The different types of generalized seizures include infantile spasms which affect young children less than five years of age, juvenile myoclonic epilepsy, typical absence seizures, atypical absence seizures, atonic seizures, tonic seizures, tonic-clonic seizures, myoclonic seizures, febrile seizures, and status epilepticus.

Infantile spasms result from developmental defects; typical absence seizures are accompanied with a very brief loss of consciousness, no convulsions and the patient simply stops their current activity with no recollection that they have even had a seizure. These types of seizures are most common among children and are they are genetically inherited.

Atypical absence seizures occur usually in patients that have Lennox-Gastaut syndrome which is a severe form of epilepsy. These seizures also occur among young children, they have a longer duration, lower pronounced loss of consciousness and more dramatic jerking than a typical absence seizure. Atonic seizures also present in children as part of Lennox-Gastaut syndrome. Children experiencing these types of seizures will fall to the ground and short-lived complete loss of both muscle tone and consciousness occur.

Tonic seizures occur usually in children while they are asleep. This type of seizure lasts about ten to fifteen seconds. They can be primarily or secondarily generalized. In the primarily generalized form, the patient calls out, falls and loses consciousness. The muscles of the head, extremities, and legs then rapidly begin contracting and relaxing. There is also occasional tongue biting, frothing of the mouth, and urinary and fecal incontinence. The secondary forms of these seizures start with a complex partial or simple partial seizure.

Myoclonic seizures are short-lived seizures. Single limbs, several limbs or the trunk can begin quick jerking motions during these seizures which are not usually accompanied with a loss of consciousness unless they evolve into generalized tonic-clonic seizures. Juvenile myoclonic epilepsy is an epilepsy syndrome which normally presents in adolescents and it can manifest with myoclonic, tonic-clonic and absence seizures.

Febrile seizures are considered a type of provoked seizure, which occur when the patient has a fever but are not affected with an intracranial infection. The two types of these seizures are benign and complicated. The patient experiences a short, solitary and generalized seizure that is tonic-clonic in appearance with the benign type; and the complicated form of these seizures can last more than fifteen minutes or recur two or more times in a twenty-four hour period.

Status epilepticus is a life-threatening condition. This condition is characterized by unrelenting persistent seizure activity without regaining consciousness between the seizures. It is a medical emergency.

A partial seizure, also referred to as a focal seizure, is subcategorized as simple partial seizures, epilepsia partialis continua which is rare, and complex partial seizures. During a simple partial seizure, the patient is conscious, but experiences motor, sensory or psychomotor symptoms.

An epilepsia partialis continuum entails focal motor seizures involving the hand, arm or one side of the face.

Complex partial seizures are often accompanied by a patient trance or stare; the person remains conscious during the seizure, but it is somewhat impaired. Motor system alterations occur with things like lip smacking, hand jerking, and uncontrollable leg movements.

The majority of seizures tend to last between thirty seconds to two minutes. Any seizure lasting for more than five minutes is considered an emergency condition. If a victim has several seizures and/or does not regain consciousness it is also considered to be an emergency.

As discussed above, there are a wide variety of signs and symptoms associated with seizure activity. Some of the most commonly occurring signs and symptoms include staring, loss of bladder control, loss of bowel control, confusion, loss of consciousness, repeated jerking of the limb(s), convulsions, lip smacking, hand rubbing, perceiving an odd smell, sound or taste, picking at clothes, drowsiness, altered responsiveness, and visual spots.

Treatments are determined on a case by case manner; the ultimate goal is to address the cause of the seizure(s.) There are several different types of medications available for the treatment of seizure disorders including Ativan, Cerebyx, Dilantin, Luminal, Depakote, and Topamax; surgery is indicated when the patient is not responding to medications and the cerebral area that is affected is small and localized. Patients who are diagnosed with seizure disorders should be encouraged to wear a medical alert bracelet and also to get adequate rest and avoid all possible seizure triggers.

HYDROCEPHALUS

Hydrocephalus is a collection of cerebrospinal fluid (CSF) in the brain. This collection creates excessive intracranial pressure which can be life threatening. Brain herniation and death occurs when intracranial pressure increases without successful treatment. The normal intracranial pressure (ICP) ranges from 5 to 15 mmHg. Hydrocephalus may be acquired or congenital. The former is primarily associated with trauma like a closed head injury or an infection; the latter is the result of some abnormal development during gestation or a genetic defect. Hydrocephalus can also be classified as communicating and non-communicating or obstructive hydrocephalus.

During infancy the skull has some limited ability to accommodate for excessive fluid because the sutures of the skull have not yet closed, however, this is not the case when the child grows older. The signs and symptoms among infants include an increase in the head circumference, irritability, lethargy, vomiting, seizures and a downward positioning of the eyes which is referred to as sun setting. Symptoms among older children and adults include nausea, vomiting, headache followed by blurred or double vision, sun setting, poor coordination, gait disturbance, urinary incontinence, developmental delays, lethargy, drowsiness, irritability, or other changes in personality or cognition including memory loss. Some of the commonly occurring other respiratory signs and symptoms include Cushing's and Cheyne-Stokes respirations. Cushing's reflex indicates that brainstem ischemia is present; and it is characterized by bradycardia, a widening pulse pressure and hypertension.

The diagnostic tests include brain scans, MRIs, a spinal tap, intracranial pressure monitoring and a gamut of neuropsychological tests.

The goal of treatment is the preservation of life and the prevention of permanent disorders. Some of the medications that are used include corticosteroids to reduce edema, intravenous osmotic diuretics, like mannitol, to remove fluid, and anticonvulsant medications to prevent seizures. A barbiturate coma is sometimes induced to lower the metabolic demands of the brain and to prevent further brain damage. Additionally, artificial ventilation is often needed; and surgical interventions are sometimes indicated to eliminate the cause of the ICP and to divert the fluid with a shunt from the CNS to another part of the body.

IMMUNOCOMPROMISE

Immunodeficiency and immunocompromise render patients unable to fight infectious diseases in a normal manner. The elements in the chain of infection include the agent, the reservoir, the environment, the mode of transmission, the portal of entry, the portal of exist and the susceptible host. Immunocompromise makes the host, or patient, highly susceptible to infections. Other factors that impact on the individual's susceptibility to infections include:

- Age: Infants and older adults are at greatest risk.

- Heredity: Many genetic factors increase the risk for infection and others protect the person against them.

- Level of stress: Stress increases cortisol levels and elevated cortisol levels decrease the person's resistance to infections and their responsiveness in terms of their anti-inflammatory responses.

- Nutritional status: People are more susceptible to infection when they have a poor nutritional status, particularly when they have a protein deficiency.

- Current medications and treatments: Treatments such as radiation therapy for cancer add to the person's susceptibility to infections. Medications like corticosteroids and antineoplastic cancer drugs decrease the person's immune responses, thus placing them at greater risk for infection than others without these medications and treatments.

The presence of diseases and other preexisting conditions: All diseases and disorders that decrease the person's defenses against infection increase the person's susceptibility to infections. For example, diseases and disorders such as diabetes mellitus, cancers that affect the bone marrow and blood cells like leukemia, lymphoma and multiple myeloma chronic infections like HIV and peripheral vascular disease increase the person's susceptibility to infections.

Immunocompromise can be classified as primary and secondary. Primary immunocompromise is defined as some immune system congenital defect that the person is born with like a defect with the lymphocytes or granulocytes; secondary immunocompromise is something that was acquired by the patient after birth.

Infections are the primary sign of immunocompromise. Opportunistic infections, defined as infections that are caused by a microorganism that does not ordinarily cause disease but is capable of doing so, under certain host conditions including immunosuppressive diseases and disorders.

The treatment of primary immunodeficiency, depending on the specific cause, can include antibody infusions and stem cell transplantation.

HEART FAILURE

In the past, heart failure was referred to as congestive cardiac failure (CCF.) The population at greatest risk for heart failure is the elderly; the risk increases as the patient grows older and older. Although neonates, infants and children are not at highest risk for heart failure, it does occur as the result of many factors including the presence of a congenital heart anomaly.

Heart failure, simply defined, is a failure of the heart's ability to pump sufficient oxygenated blood to meet the demands and requirements of the body's tissues. Some of the most common causes of heart failure include hypertension, congenital heart disorders, ischemic heart disease, and cardiomyopathy. It is left ventricular systolic compromise that is the most common underlying cause of heart failure, but right sided ventricular dysfunction as well as biventricular failure can also lead to heart failure.

Left ventricular failure is most commonly caused by systemic hypertension, cardiomyopathy, bacterial endocarditis, myocardial infarction, aortic stenosis, aortic regurgitation, and mitral regurgitation; right ventricular failure is most often associated with mitral stenosis, pulmonary hypertension, bacterial endocarditis, and right ventricular infarction; and biventricular heart failure is typically the result of cardiomyopathy, myocarditis, left ventricular failure, dysrhythmias, anemia, and thyrotoxicosis

Poor heart contractions manifest in terms of a number of signs and symptoms including fluid retention, dyspnea, tachycardia, fatigue, pallor, hypotension, lethargy, activity intolerance and anxiety. Pathophysiologically, renal, hemodynamic, neural, and hormonal changes can also occur as the result of heart failure.

Heart failure is treated with a number of different drugs, including diuretics to reduce fluid overload, ACE inhibitors, angiotensin II receptor antagonists when the patient cannot tolerate ACE inhibitors and beta blockers. Treatment can also include biventricular pacing, an implanted cardioverter defibrillator, restricted fluid intake, a low sodium diet and a medically approved exercise routine.

Heart Failure in Neonates

Acute heart failure during the first week of life is an ominous sign and a medical emergency. An umbilical venous catheter is used to establish vascular access, intravenous infusions of prostaglandin E1 at an initial dosage of 0.01 mcg/kg/min, or up to 0.1 as needed, are given to maintain the patency of the ductus arteriosus, and mechanical ventilation in addition to the careful use of supplemental oxygen are also common interventions. Neonates and infants receiving supplemental oxygen must be closely monitored because it can decrease pulmonary vascular resistance and jeopardize patients when they have a disorder such as hypoplastic left heart syndrome.

Other therapies for neonatal heart failure include diuretics such as furosemide, drugs to reduce afterload and inotropic drugs such as dopamine, milrinon or dobutamine, all of which can lead to cardiac arrhythmias. Postoperatively, neonates are given nitroprusside as a vasodilator to prevent hypertension.

Heart Failure in Older Infants and Children

Furosemide with an initial dosage of 0.5 to 1.0 mg/kg intravenously or 1 to 3 mg/kg orally titrated upward as needed, an ACE inhibitor like captopril and/or digoxin may be given. In addition to medications, a healthy salt restricted diet is recommended and, at times, tube feedings may be indicated.

INHALATION INJURIES

Smoke Inhalation

Smoke inhalation injures in combination with a thermal burn has a high rate of morbidity and mortality but the rates associated with only smoke inhalation are significant lower. This inhalation injury is suggested with a history of proximity to a fire and with the presence of soot and facial burns, however adventitious breath sounds such as crackles, wheezing, stridor, dyspnea and rhonchi are typically not present unless the inhalation is severe so other methods of detection and diagnosis are used.

Smoke inhalation causes impaired oxygenation and impaired ventilation which lead to a number of life threatening situations such as increases in airway resistance, the work of breathing, oxygen consumption needs, intrapulmonary shunting and dead space. It also impairs surfactant production, ciliary action and lung/chest wall compliance. Severe cases can lead to bronchospasm, hypoxemia, airway edema, airway obstruction and respiratory arrest among the pediatric and neonatal population.

The inhalation of incomplete products of combustion rather than the smoke itself causes damage to the lung parenchyma; damage to the pulmonary macrophages and respiratory epithelium leads to an inflammatory response, edema, the collection of epithelial cell debris, atelectasis, and, at times, hyaline membrane disruption. Systemically, this inhalation can lead to decrease in oxygenation, surfactant production and lung compliance in addition to increases in airway resistance, oxygen consumption and ventilation-perfusion mismatching.

Carbon Monoxide Inhalation

Smoke inhalation, in addition to its effects as discussed above, also leads to carbon monoxide inhalation and possible poisoning. Carbon monoxide poisoning can also occur when automobiles are left running in an enclosed area such as a garage and other environmental causes.

Carbon monoxide impedes the absorption of oxygen because this colorless, odorless gas binds to hemoglobin with an affinity for this binding that is 200 to 280 times greater than the affinity of oxygen to hemoglobin. Carboxyhemoglobin forms when the carbon monoxide attaches to hemoglobin thus causing a drastic reduction in the ability of the body to oxygenate.

The direct measurement of carboxyhemoglobin is done with co-oximetry rather than pulse oximetry because the later does not accurately measure oxygen saturation in the presence of carboxyhemoglobin.

The most severe effects of carbon monoxide poisoning affect the major organs and systems such as the brain, the CNS and the heart as the result of the anoxia. Other symptoms according to the percentage of carboxyhemoglobin from the lowest to the highest percentage are headache, dyspnea, blurred vision, nausea, vomiting, severe headache, tachypnea, tachycardia, confusion, depressed level of consciousness, seizures, bradycardia, respiratory failure and death.

The treatment for carbon monoxide includes administering pure oxygen through a face mask, or a ventilator, and in some cases it may be necessary for hyperbaric oxygen therapy.

Chemical Inhalation Injuries

The signs and symptoms vary according to the agent and the volume/duration of the inhalation. Some of the signs and symptoms include respiratory distress, acute airway and lung obstruction which can lead to death. Lung inflammation, bronchospasm, pulmonary edema, sloughing of tissue and scar formation can also occur in the respiratory passages and the lungs. Corrosive agents can lead to hemorrhage and permanent, irreversible scarring.

The goal of treatment for chemical inhalation injuries is to maintain adequate oxygenation. Analgesic medications, corticosteroids, oxygen, bronchodilators, humidification, and ventilator support are often indicated.

The diagnosis of smoke inhalation injuries is made with the use of:

- Fiber optic bronchoscopy to visualize the airway and the extent of the injury

- Xenon scanning to determine the amount of parenchymal damage

- Spirometry

- Thermal and dye dilution evaluations to determine the amount of extravascular lung fluid and to differentiate between parenchymal lung damage and upper airway damage

Spirometry, when done among members of the pediatric population within 24 hours after the injury, will reveal a decrease in the forced expiratory volume in 1 second as well as the ratio of FEV1 to vital capacity.

The goal of treatment for inhalation injuries is to restore and maintain adequate respiratory functioning while decreasing the risk of any complications. The treatments, depending on the severity, include:

- Oxygen therapy with 100% oxygen

- Bronchial hygiene therapy including coughing, chest physiotherapy, therapeutic bronchoscopy, early ambulation and suctioning

- Airway maintenance using an artificial airway

- Pharmacologic interventions

- Mechanical ventilator support when indicated

Some of the pharmacological agents that are used include B2 agonists to treat and prevent bronchospasm, aerosolized racemic epinephrine to serve as a bronchodilator and a vasoconstrictor to reduce edema, corticosteroids to decrease the inflammatory response and edema and maintain surfactant function, N-acetyl cysteine and heparin in combination to prevent atelectasis and other complications associated with inhalation injuries. Prophylactic antibiotics are not indicated until there is a confirmatory culture for a bacterial infection such as pneumonia.

Based on the fact that inhalation injury victims are at risk for ventilator-use lung damage, mechanical ventilation is used cautiously and only when necessary to sustain life. When conventional mechanical ventilation is indicated it is usually initiated with a tidal volume of 6 to 8 mL/kg, although it should be carefully considered determined as based on the patient's level of oxygenation, lung/thorax compliance, resistance and other considerations. PEEP improves oxygenation and to increase mean airway pressures. PEEP varies according to the severity of the damage and it is often increased with very severe smoke inhalation injuries.

PRACTICE EXAM 1

1. You will have three hours to complete the exam.
2. The exam consists of 140* multiple choice questions. 120 will be scored and 20 are for future use.

*This practice test consists of 150 multiple choice practice questions.

PRACTICE EXAMINATION

1. The four basic methods or techniques that are used for physical assessment are:

   a) Inspection, palliation, percussion, and distillation.
   b) Concentration, palpitation, percussion, and application.
   c) Percussion, auscultation, palpation, and inspection.
   d) Auscultation, palpitation, inspection, and percussion.

2. Select the component of a thorough physical assessment that is accurately paired with its assessment element(s.)

   a) Pulses: Rate, volume, moderation, rhythm, resonance and equality.
   b) Skin assessment: Elasticity, temperature and the presence of any lesions.
   c) Pulse pressure: The mathematical stability of the systolic and diastolic blood pressures.
   d) Diaphragmatic movement: The palpation of the lungs and breath sounds.

3. The S1 sound:

   a) Starts when systole begins and it is mostly from tricuspid valve closure.
   b) May be very high-pitched and piercing with mitral regurgitation.
   c) May be low-pitched and nearly inaudible with mitral stenosis.
   d) Starts when systole begins and it results from primarily mitral valve closure.

4. Your patient has a murmur that is loud and audible with minimal stethoscope to chest contact. What grade is this murmur?

   a) Grade 2
   b) Grade 3
   c) Grade 4
   d) Grade 5

5. **Select the type of murmur that is accurately paired with its possible causes.**

   a) Mid to late systolic murmur: Obstruction of the aorta or the Tetralogy of Fallot
   b) Holosystolic murmur: Ventral septal defect or regurgitation of the tricuspid valve
   c) Mid diastolic murmur: Pulmonic obstruction or papillary muscle impairment
   d) Early diastolic regurgitant murmur: Mitral valve prolapse or obstruction of the aorta

6. **You are going to assess your patient's peripheral vascular system. What assessment techniques will you employ?**

   a) Observing the patient's skin temperature and examining the carotid pulse
   b) Palpating the temporal artery and examining the basilic veins
   c) Listening to all bilateral pulses and checking the skin color
   d) Auscultating the carotid pulse and inspecting the patient's jugular veins.

7. **Select the cranial nerve that is accurately paired with its description.**

   a) Optic: Regulates most eye movements
   b) Trochlear: Controls facial expressions
   c) Acoustic: Provides the ability to sense gravity
   d) Facial: Allows eye abduction

8. **A normal white blood count is:**

   a) 4.2 to 5.4 million cells/mcL
   b) 4.7 to 6.1 million cells/mcL
   c) 4,500 to 10,000 cells/mcL
   d) 4,000 to 10,500 cells/mcL

9. **Your patient is affected with a gram positive bacteria. Which bacteria is this patient most likely affected with?**

   a) Escherichia coli
   b) Pseudomonas
   c) Klebsiella

d) Enterococcus

10. Select the electrolyte that is accurately paired with its normal range.

   a) Chloride: 95 to 106 mEq/L
   b) Bicarbonate: 25 to 32 mEq/L
   c) Calcium: 2.5 to 4.5 mEq/L
   d) Glucose: 160 to 210 mg/100 mL

11. What percentage and category of impairment is present following bronchodilator therapy when the current test identified a pulmonary function impairment of 50%?

   a) 51% or higher and in the mild to normal range
   b) 64% or higher and in the mild to normal range
   c) 50% to 64% and in the mild to normal range
   d) 64% to 79% and in the mild to normal range.

12. Select the disorder accurately paired with its ABG value.

   a) Pneumonia: pH 7.52, PaCO2 27 torr, PaO2 48 torr, HCO3 22mEq/L and BE-1
   b) Pneumonia: pH 7.52, PaCO2 58 torr, PaO2 48 torr, HCO3 22mEq/L and BE +0.7
   c) Pulmonary emboli: pH 7.36, PaCO2 58 torr, PaO2 48 torr, HCO3 22mEq/L and BE -1
   d) Pulmonary emboli: pH 7.52, PaCO2 58 torr, PaO2 48 torr, HCO3 22mEq/L and BE +0.7

13. Which is a benefit of CT angiography when contrasted to conventional angiography?

   a) It is preferred for the detection of tumors and cysts.
   b) It is less invasive and provides high levels of accuracy.
   c) It provides superior images of the vascular structures.
   d) It can be used to describe the metabolism of the heart.

14. **Your patient is being scheduled for PET scanning and V/Q scanning. As the respiratory therapist, you are teaching the patient and their family members about these nuclear scanning tests. Which of the following statements should be included in this patient teaching?**

   a) V/Q scanning uses fluorodeoxyglucose to assess and measure the metabolic activity in tissues and to determine pulmonary perfusion and ventilation.
   b) V/Q scanning uses intravenous administration of radioactive technetium and is indicated when an under perfusion of the pulmonary circulation is suspected.
   c) PET scanning uses fluorodeoxyglucose to examine the metabolic activity in tissues and to determine the size and extent of a myocardial infarction.
   d) PET scanning uses intravenous administration of intravenous radionuclide and identifies the rapid metabolic rate of cells like those linked with lung cancer.

15. **Select the age group that is correctly paired with its normal respiratory rate.**

   a) People from 17 to 65 years of age: 12-16 breaths per minute
   b) Toddlers from 1 to 2 years of age: 30-60 breaths per minute
   c) Preschool children from 3 to 5 years of age: 22-34 breaths per minute
   d) School-age children from 6 to 12 years of age: 24-40 breaths per minute

16. **The method for calculating the I:E ratio is:**

   a) Ti (Te)
   b) Ti / Te
   c) (Ti / Te)2
   d) Ti (Te)2

17. **You are conducting an in-service class for new RTs relating to respiratory care. One of the teaching sessions includes information about residual volumes and forced inspiratory volume. Which information would you include in this class?**

    a) Residual volume is the amount of gas that can be exhaled at the end of a forceful expiratory phase.
    b) Residual volume is the amount of gas left in the lung at the end of a forceful expiratory phase.
    c) Forced Inspiratory volume is the greatest amount of gas that can be inhaled from the end of the inspiratory phase.
    d) Forced Inspiratory volume is the greatest amount of gas that can be inhaled from the end of the expiratory phase.

18. **Which equation is used to calculate the ratio of dead space over tidal volume?**

    a) PaCO2-PeCO2(PaCO2)
    b) PeCO2-PaCO2(PaCO2)
    c) PaCO2-PeCO2/PaCO2
    d) PeCO2-PaCO2/PaCO2

19. **Arterial blood gas results can indicate:**

    a) The presence of any condition associated with moderate to severe hypoxemia such as a pulmonary embolus.
    b) A CO2 balance or imbalance in the extra-cellular fluid and how much carbon monoxide removal occurs during breathing.
    c) A higher than normal diffusion capacity as associated with pulmonary fibrosis and emphysema.
    d) A combination of restrictive and obstructive lung disorders like cystic fibrosis or pulmonary fibrosis.

20. **Which of the following statements about hypercapnia or hypocapnia is accurate?**

    a) Hypercapnia is associated with carbon monoxide poisoning from automobiles and smoke inhalation from smoking.
    b) Hypocapnia if defined as Pco2 less than 35 mm Hg and hypercapnia is defined as Pco2 of greater than 45 mm Hg.
    c) Hypercapnia if defined as Pco2 greater than 35 mm Hg and hypocapnia is defined as Pco2 of less than 25 mm Hg.

d) Hypocapnia is associated with pulmonary abnormalities such as an inability to increase ventilation and a febrile state.

21. Select the age group that is correctly paired with its normal resting cardiac rate.

    a) Infants and neonates: 120 to 140 BPM
    b) Young children from 1 to 10 years of age: 70 to 120 BPM
    c) Adults from age 17 to 55 years of age: 60 to 90 BPM
    d) Adults from age 56 years of age and up: 40 to 70 BPM

22. Which hemodynamic monitoring value should cause concern for the respiratory therapists?

    a) A mixed venous oxygen saturation of 60% to 80%
    b) A right atrium pressure of 10 to 80 mm Hg
    c) A left Ventricle end diastolic of 15 to 22 mm Hg
    d) A brachial artery mean of 7 to 15 mm Hg

23. The Fick method is based on the premise that cardiac output is:

    a) Disproportionate to oxygen consumption divided by the arteriovenous oxygen difference.
    b) Proportionate to oxygen consumption multiplied by the arteriovenous oxygen difference.
    c) Disproportionate to oxygen consumption multiplied by the arteriovenous oxygen difference.
    d) Proportionate to oxygen consumption divided by the arteriovenous oxygen difference.

24. An L/S ratio:

    a) Greater than 1:1 before the 35th week of gestation signals a high risk for respiratory distress syndrome.
    b) Less than 2:1 after the 35th week of gestation is normal and an indicator of proper lung development.
    c) 2:1 by the 35th week of gestation is normal and an indicator of normal lung development.
    d) Of 2:1 or greater after the 36th week of gestation may indicate hyaline membrane disease.

25. Select the normal neonatal vital sign range.

a) Respirations from 40 to 70 per minute
b) Pulse from 100 to 160 BPM
c) Blood pressure: Diastolic from 40 to 50 mm Hg and systolic from 60 to 70 mm Hg
d) Temperature range from 98.9 to 100.9 degrees

26. The neonate experiencing respiratory apnea pauses breathing for a duration of at least:

a) 15 seconds.
b) 12 seconds.
c) 10 seconds.
d) 5 seconds.

27. Which of the following assessments indicates normal neonatal growth and development?

a) Weight of 2,000 to 3,200 g
b) Length of 50 to 60 cm
c) Head circumference of 30 to 33 cm
d) Chest circumference of 30 to 33 cm

28. Select the neonate's weight classification that is correctly paired with its description.

a) Low birth weight: Weighs less than 2,500 g at the time of delivery.
b) Appropriate for gestational age: 40th to the 60th percentile.
c) Large for gestational age: The neonate's weight is above the 75th percentile.
d) Small for gestational age: The neonate's weight is below the 25th percentile.

29. Which of the following is an accurate description of possible findings when using the trans-illumination procedure on a premature infant?

a) Malignant tumors will appear as light red or pink in color.
b) Hydrocele will appear as black or dark brown in color.
c) Internal bleeding will appear very dark or black in color.
d) Pneumothorax appears as very violet or purple in color.

30. Tracheal deviation can include:

a) Empyema when the trachea is toward the affected side.
b) Pulmonary fibrosis when trachea is away from affected side.
c) Tension pneumothorax when trachea is toward affected side.
d) Atelectasis when trachea is toward affected side.

31. Which set of CPAP and BIPAP titration procedures are done to determine the patient's correct pressure in order to stop episodes of hypopnea or apnea?

a) Pressure is set at 3 to 4 cm to begin, increased by 1-2 cm every 5 to 15 minutes until 10 cm, then by 0.5 cm every 5 to 15 minutes, until episodes of hypopnea or apnea no longer occur.
b) Pressure is set at 2 to 3 cm to begin, increased by 2-3 cm every 5 to 15 minutes until 10 cm, then by 0.5-1.5 cm every 5 to 15 minutes, until episodes of hypopnea or apnea no longer occur.
c) Pressure is set at 3 to 4 cm to begin, increased by 1-2 cm every 5 to 15 minutes until 10 cm, then by 0.5 cm every 15 to 30 minutes, until episodes of hypopnea or apnea no longer occur.
d) Pressure is set at 2 to 3 cm to begin, increased by 2-3 cm every 15 to 30 minutes until 10 cm, then by 0.5 cm every 15 to 30 minutes, until episodes of hypopnea or apnea no longer occur.

32. What is the correct sequence initiating bilevel ventilation?

a) Setting the expiratory positive pressure, adjusting the inspiratory positive airway pressure, adjusting the expiratory positive pressure to achieve the desired tidal volume, and setting the inspiratory positive airway pressure.
b) Setting the expiratory positive pressure, adjusting the expiratory positive pressure to achieve the desired tidal volume, setting the inspiratory positive airway pressure, and adjusting the inspiratory positive airway pressure.
c) Setting the inspiratory positive airway pressure, setting the expiratory positive pressure, adjusting the expiratory positive pressure to achieve the desired tidal volume, and adjusting the inspiratory positive airway pressure.
d) Setting the expiratory positive pressure, setting the inspiratory positive airway pressure, adjusting the inspiratory positive airway pressure, and adjusting the

expiratory positive pressure to achieve the desired tidal volume.

33. Select the age group that is accurately paired with the recommended sizes of suction catheters.

a) Pediatric patients from 18 months to 8 years of age: 6 to 8 Fr
b) Pediatric patients from 18 months to 8 years of age: 10 to 12 Fr
c) Pediatric patients from 18 months to 8 years of age: 8 to 10 Fr
d) Pediatric patients from 18 months to 8 years of age: 4 to 6 Fr

34. External humidification systems are not needed when a:

a) A compressor utilizing sodium aluminum silicate filtering is used.
b) A semipermeable plastic membrane oxygen concentrator is used.
c) A molecular sieve oxygen concentrated system is used.
d) A molecular sieve sodium concentrated filtering system is used.

35. The inflexible vest used during high frequency chest wall oscillation effectively increases the clearance of tracheal mucous by deflating and inflating on the patient's chest about every:

a) 10 to 15 times per minute.
b) 15 to 20 times per minute.
c) 5 to 10 times per second.
d) 5 to 20 times per second.

36. Which mechanical ventilation intervention can prevent ventilator associated pneumonia?

a) Maintaining cuff pressure in the endotracheal tube at 30-40 mmHg
b) Changing heat and moisture exchangers at least every 24-36 hours
c) Elevation of the head of the bed from 20 to 25 degrees unless contraindicated
d) Providing oral care with 2% chlorhexidine and water-soluble mouth moisturizer

37. **What is the correct equation for calculating airway resistance?**

   a) $\dfrac{\text{Peak airway pressure} - \text{Peak flow in liters/sec}}{\text{Plateau pressure}}$

   b) $\dfrac{\text{Peak airway pressure} - \text{Plateau pressure}}{\text{Peak flow in liters/sec}}$

   c) $\dfrac{\text{Plateau pressure} - \text{Peak flow in liters/sec}}{\text{Peak airway pressure}}$

   d) $\dfrac{\text{Peak flow in liters/sec} - \text{Plateau pressure}}{\text{Peak airway pressure}}$

38. **What color coding should a cylinder containing carbon dioxide and oxygen have?**

   a) Brown and green
   b) Brown and white
   c) Gray and green
   d) Gray and white

39. **You are asked to transport a patient who is receiving oxygen from a nasal cannula at 6 L/min. The pressure gauge on the cylinder reads 1200 psi. How long will the cylinder provide the appropriate oxygen flow?**

   a) 94 minutes
   b) 69 minutes
   c) 112 minutes
   d) 74 minutes

40. **A patient has been connected to a portable vacuum system due to the central vacuum system undergoing maintenance. You discover the equipment is not functioning correctly. What trouble shooting can you do before replacing the unit?**

   a) Check to make sure that the unit is plugged into an outlet and that it is turned on and set to the desired positive pressure.
   b) Change the collection bottle, empty or not, and replace all the tubing with new tubing and check for any leaking.
   c) Make sure there tubing is correctly coiled to avoid accidental tripping or stepping on it and that the collection bottle is not full.

d) Check to see if the system is turned on and set to the desired negative pressure and that all connected tubing is sealed with no leaks.

41. Which type of ventilator is most often utilized in a NICU?

a) Microprocessor
b) Fluidic
c) Pneumatic
d) Electrical

42. Select the age group that is correctly paired with its medication consideration.

a) Elderly: Adult dosage to begin and then reductions of 25-30% thereafter.
b) Toddler: Dosages based on body weight and measured in kilograms.
c) Preschool and school age children: 30-50% of a normal adult dosage.
d) Adolescent: 50% of adult dosage to begin and then increases of 25% thereafter.

43. If a catheter is a 7 Fr, what are the outer and inner diameters?

a) Outer= 3.12 cm, inner= 2.15 cm
b) Outer= 3.21 cm, inner= 2.51 cm
c) Outer= 2.13 cm, inner= 1.52 cm
d) Outer= 2.31 cm, inner= 1.25 cm

44. Select the respiratory medication that is accurately paired with its correct description.

a) Bronchodilators are used to treat airway bleeding and edema by decreasing ciliary motility and encouraging the release of histamine.
b) Cromolyn sodium is used to treat chronic asthma, however it is not recommended as prevention for exercise induced asthma.
c) Leukotriene is contraindicated among children less than 15 years of age and children or adults that are affected with liver disease.

d) Mucolytic are used to deter secretion mobilization and have gained popularity as a respiratory treatment option in many healthcare settings.

45. An example of a depolarizing neuromuscular blocker is:

a) Gallamine trethiodide
b) Pancuronium
c) Attacurium besylate
d) Succinylcholine chloride

46. Select the abnormal breathing pattern that is correctly paired with its probable cause.

a) Friction rubs: A pulmonary infarct
b) Kussmaul respirations: Acute epiglottitis
c) Biot respirations: Metabolic acidosis
d) Cheyne-Stokes Respirations: Pneumonia

47. Select the statement about broncho-provocation studies that is accurately paired with its description.

a) Nebulized treatments are repeated at specific time increments and spirometry testing is completed after each treatment to assess any increase in FEV1.
b) Broncho-provocation tests are indicated whenever a patient is affected with a cardiac, neurological and/or pulmonary disorder such as an aortic aneurysm.
c) A positive spirometry tests before or after a nebulized treatment with a decrease in the FEV1 of 20% below the baseline is suggestive of asthma.
d) Some of the inhalation medications and substances used in broncho-provocation tests include cold air, histamine, sodium benzoate, and methacholin.

48. To properly drain the apical bronchus of the lingula, the patient should be put into a:

a) 45 degree Trendelenburg position and turned on the right side.
b) Prone position with a pillow under the hip.
c) Semi-Fowler's position and leaning to the right, to the left and then forward.
d) Supine position with a pillow under the knees.

49. The cuff pressure for an endotracheal tube should be maintained at what?

    a) 15 and 20 mm Hg
    b) 15 and 25 mm Hg
    c) 20 and 25 mm Hg
    d) 20 and 30 mm Hg

50. The five stages of Roger's Innovation-Decision Process are:

    a) Knowledge, persuasion, decision, implementation and confirmation.
    b) Knowledge, persuasion, decision, application and confirmation.
    c) Knowledge, persuasion, conclusion, implementation and confirmation.
    d) Knowledge, persuasion, conclusion, application and confirmation.

51. You are caring for an infant in the emergency department who has presented with the mother. The 1 month old infant is diagnosed with apnea. As you begin to interview the mother about her maternal history, the mother states, "It does not matter how many pregnancies and live births I have had. I am here because my baby has stopped breathing." How should you respond to this comment?

    a) "I fully understand your concern about the baby but it is the policy of this emergency department to interview all new mothers about their maternal history."
    b) "You are correct. Our greatest concern is your baby and not your maternal history."
    c) "Maternal history is an important and significant part of the baby's assessment especially during infancy."
    d) "I will ask the doctor to see you and explain why this maternal history is so important to us in the emergency department."

52. **You have just been paged to go to the maternity area because an infant who has aspirated meconium before birth. Your rapid assessment of this neonate is that the newborn is vigorous. What intervention(s) should you be prepared to perform or assist with?**

   a) Normal neonate resuscitation procedures
   b) Intubation
   c) Intubation and suctioning
   d) Bronchoscopy

53. **A self-inflating resuscitation bag is highly beneficial in the neonatal area because it is:**

   a) Capable of delivering 100% oxygen.
   b) Capable of delivering free flow oxygen.
   c) Readily attachable to a T piece.
   d) Portable and accessible.

54. **Which factors are assessed in order to determine gestational age?**

   a) Ballard scoring, weight and chest circumference
   b) Bollard scoring, Apgar scoring and chest circumference
   c) Apgar scoring, chest circumference and weight
   d) Pulse oximetry, laboratory results and weight

55. **Select the hemodynamic measurement that is accurately paired with its normal value.**

   a) Pulmonary Artery Peak Systolic: 15 to 30 mm Hg
   b) Pulmonary Artery End Diastolic: 15 to 30 mm Hg
   c) Left Atrium A Wave: 6 to 12 mm Hg
   d) Left Atrium V Wave: 4 to 16 mm Hg

56. You have auscultated a young child's breath sounds. You hear breath sounds between the scapulae and the 1st and second intercostals spaces during both expiration and inspiration. The father of the child asks you how the child's lungs are. How should you respond to this father's question?

   a) "I heard an abnormal breath sound that could mean that your child has an infection like a flu."
   b) "I heard an abnormal breath sound that could mean that your child a cold."
   c) "I heard a normal breath sound when your child inhaled and exhaled."
   d) "I heard a normal breath sound when your child inhaled but it was abnormal when he exhaled."

57. Which of the following is an adventitious breath sound that can be relieved with coughing?

   a) Rales
   b) Rhonchi
   c) Wheezing
   d) Friction rub

58. You are assessing the infant's heart sounds and you hear a click at the beginning of S_1. How would you interpret this click?

   a) You would recognize that this is a normal heart sound for neonates and infants.
   b) You would recognize that this heart sound will resolve itself by the time the child is 1 year old.
   c) You would recognize that this abnormal heart sound suggests the presence of aortic stenosis.
   d) You would recognize that this abnormal heart sound suggests the presence of left bundle branch block.

59. Which cardiac arrhythmia is most common among patients affected with a pulmonary embolus?

   a) Atrial fibrillation
   b) First-degree atrioventricular block
   c) Atrial flutter
   d) Second-degree atrioventricular block

60. **As you are assessing an infant, you notice that the infant manifests a "walk" like movement of the feet when the infant's soles touch the floor when you place them there. How would you interpret this assessment finding?**

    a) This is an abnormal assessment finding and it could indicate the presence of spina bifida.
    b) This is an abnormal assessment finding and it could indicate the presence of muscular dystrophy.
    c) This is a normal assessment finding. The child is demonstrating the truncal incurvation reflex.
    d) This is a normal assessment finding. The child is demonstrating the step reflex.

61. **The adequate mean blood pressure (MBP) is calculated with which formula?**

    a) Adequate MBP = Gestational age in weeks plus 5
    b) Adequate MBP = Gestational age in weeks plus 10
    c) Adequate MBP = I: E ratio plus the number of weeks of gestation
    d) Adequate MBP = V: Q ratio plus the number of weeks of gestation

62. **Which scoring system is used for the assessment of neonatal respiratory distress?**

    a) The Silverman scoring system
    b) The Apgar scoring system
    c) The Coombs' scoring system
    d) The Neilson scoring system

63. **What is the normal level of C reactive protein?**

    a) From 1.0 to 10 mg/dL
    b) From 2.0 to 10 mg/dL
    c) < 1.0 mg/dL
    d) > 1.0 mg/dL

64. **The proper size of an oropharyngeal airway is determined by measuring the distance from:**

    a) The external pinna to the mouth.
    b) The angle of the jaw to the external pinna.
    c) The external pinna to the nares.
    d) The angle of the jaw to the mouth.

65. **Select the phase of the respiratory cycle that is paired with its definition.**

    a) Phase I: The transition inspiration to expiration
    b) Phase II: Expiration
    c) Phase III: The transition from inspiration to expiration
    d) Phase IV: Inhalation

66. **You are caring for a patient who has asthma and an irritable airway. Which airway is indicated for this patient?**

    a) A laryngeal mask
    b) An endotracheal tube
    c) A corrugated tube
    d) A positive pressure tube

67. **You are caring for a 3 year old who has Treacher Collins syndrome and is in need of intubation. Which type of laryngoscope do you expect will be used for this intubation?**

    a) An alligator laryngoscope
    b) A Holinger laryngoscope
    c) A Pierre Robin laryngoscope
    d) A Holter laryngoscope

68. **The depth of an endotracheal tube in cm is calculated with which formula?**

    a) The depth of the endotracheal tube in cm = 15 + Age in Years + 1
    b) The depth of the endotracheal tube in cm = 10 + Age in Years + 3
    c) The depth of the endotracheal tube in cm = 15 + Age in Years + 3
    d) The depth of the endotracheal tube in cm = 10 + Age in Years + 1

69. What does the "I" of the MSMAID mnemonic represent?

   a) Intubation
   b) Inhalation
   c) Inspection
   d) Intravenous

70. You are preparing an in-service class for nurses relating to respiratory care and volumes. Which definition should you include in this teaching?

   a) Expiratory reserve volume is the greatest amount of air that can be exhaled after the end expiratory phase.
   b) Expiratory reserve volume is the greatest amount of air that can be inhaled after the end expiratory phase.
   c) Residual volume is the amount of oxygen left in the lung at the end of a forceful exhalation.
   d) Residual volume is the amount of oxygen left in the lung at the end of a forceful inhalation.

71. You are ready to suction a 4 year old child. What size suction catheter should you use?

   a) 5 Fr
   b) 6 Fr
   c) 8 Fr
   d) 12 Fr

72. What color is used for a helium canister?

   a) White
   b) Yellow
   c) Black
   d) Brown

73. Select the oxygen delivery device that is accurately paired with its description.

   a) Partial Rebreathing Reservoir Mask: 2 to 15L/min is usually enough to maintain the FIO2 up to 0.6
   b) Partial Rebreathing Reservoir Mask: 6 to 15L/min is usually enough to maintain the FIO2 up to 0.6
   c) High Flow Nasal Cannula: A maximum of 4 L/min
   d) High Flow Nasal Cannula: A maximum of 5 L/min

74. **Select the mode of ventilation that is accurately paired with its description.**

    a) Bilevel positive airway pressure (BiPAP): Preset positive pressure only during spontaneous inspiration
    b) Bilevel positive airway pressure (BiPAP): Preset positive pressure only during spontaneous
    c) expiration
    d) High frequency ventilation: Contraindicated for pediatric patients
    e) Inverse ratio ventilation: Lengthens inspiratory phase

75. **The airway resistance is mathematically calculated using which formula?**

    a) Airway resistance = $\dfrac{\text{Peak flow in L/min}}{60 \text{ seconds}}$

    b) Airway resistance = $\dfrac{\text{Peak flow in L/min}}{\text{Peak flow in liters/sec}}$

    c) Airway resistance = $\dfrac{\text{Peak airway pressure} - \text{End pressure}}{\text{Peak flow in liters/sec}}$

    d) Airway resistance = $\dfrac{\text{Peak airway pressure} - \text{Plateau pressure}}{\text{Peak flow in liters/sec}}$

76. **You are teaching the mother of a young child about extracorporeal life support. Which content should be included in the teaching plan?**

    a) Extracorporeal life support circuits exchange gases across a membrane.
    b) Extracorporeal life support circuits consist of a helium mixture.
    c) Extracorporeal life support circuits contain a nitric oxide gas.
    d) Extracorporeal life support circuits have a driving pressure of oxygen at 45mm Hg.

77. Extracorporeal membrane oxygenation (ECMO) is indicated when the pediatric patient is:

    a) Less than 34 weeks of gestation.
    b) Less than 2 kg in weight.
    c) Affected with a congenital diaphragmatic hernia.
    d) Affected with a non-cyanotic congenital heart disorder.

78. The formula to determine the desired FIO2 is:

    a) $\text{Desired FiO}_2 = \dfrac{\text{Current FiO}_2 \times \text{Desired PaO}_2}{\text{Current PaCO}_2}$

    b) $\text{Desired FiO}_2 = \dfrac{\text{Current FiO}_2 \times \text{Desired PaO}_2}{\text{Current PaO}_2}$

    c) $\text{Desired FiO}_2 = \dfrac{\text{Current FiO}_2 \times \text{Desired PaCO}_2}{\text{Current PaO}_2}$

    d) $\text{Desired FiO}_2 = \dfrac{\text{Current FiO}_2 \times \text{Desired PaO}_2}{\text{Current FiO}_2}$

79. Which mode of ventilation would you recommend when you want to enable the patient to trigger off tidal volume despite the fact that there is a preset interval?

    a) Control ventilation
    b) Intermittent mandatory ventilation
    c) Synchronous intermittent mandatory ventilation
    d) Expiratory reserve ventilation

80. Which of the following is a method of weaning a patient off a ventilator?

    a) Intermittent ventilator discontinuance
    b) Synchronous IMV weaning
    c) Asynchronous IMV weaning
    d) Intermittent IMV weaning

81. Which patient is at greatest risk for retrolental fibroplasias as the result of oxygen supplementation?

    a) A 16 month old infant
    b) A 6 month old premature infant
    c) A child with cystic fibrosis
    d) A newborn premature infant

87. This helps prevent ventilator-associated pneumonia:

a) Oral care with lidocaine
b) Oral care with a lactose solution
c) A supine position
d) A semi-Fowler's position

88. Who will benefit from high frequency chest wall oscillation?

a) A pediatric patient with cystic fibrosis
b) A pediatric patient with pneumonia
c) An elderly patient with pneumonia
d) An elderly patient with COPD

89. What level of humidity does ANSI and the American Association for Respiratory Care recommend?

a) ≥30 mg H2O/L
b) 10 to 30 mg H2O/L
c) 20 to 60 mg H2O/L
d) 5 to 10 mg H2O/L

90. The AARC established the need for supplemental humidity for all oxygen flows of more than:

a) 1 L/min.
b) 2 L/min.
c) 3 L/min.
d) 4 L/min.

91. Nitric oxide therapy is used for respiratory disorders such as:

a) Persistent pulmonary hypertension of the neonate
b) Croup
c) Bronchiolitis
d) Apnea

92. Which law of physics states that volume is inversely proportionate to pressure?

a) Boyle's law
b) Dalton's law
c) Poiseuille's law
d) Graham's law

93. The usual pediatric dosage of intravenous midazolam is from:

a) 0.05 mg/kg to 0.3 mg/kg with a max dosage of 0.4 to 0.6 mg/kg.
b) 1 ug/kg to 3 ug/kg with a max dosage of no more than 5-10 ug/kg.
c) 0.05 mg to 0.3 mg with a max dosage of 0.4 to 0.6 mg.
d) 1 ug to 3 ug with a max dosage of no more than 5 to 10 ug.

94. What respiratory effect can your patient experience on a plane (fixed-wing) as it ascends to flight altitude?

a) Increased barometric pressure
b) The fraction of inspired oxygen increases
c) A reduction in the delivery of oxygen
d) Endotracheal cuff deflation

95. Which law of physics states that the pressure of gas mixtures is equal to the sum of the partial pressures of the gases that make up the mixture of gases?

a) Boyle's law
b) Dalton's law
c) Poiseuille's law
d) Graham's law

96. Your patient's doctor has asked you to prepare for the insertion of a peripheral artery catheter for your patient. Which site will you most likely prepare for this catheter?

a) The jugular artery
b) The radial artery
c) The external iliac artery
d) The internal iliac artery

97. The length of an umbilical artery catheter is:

a) At least 16 inches.
b) More than 16 inches.
c) Referenced on a nomogram as based on the distance from the umbilicus to the shoulder.
d) Is equal to the distance from the umbilicus to the shoulder.

98. Which Swan-Ganz catheter port will you use to measure pulmonary capillary wedge pressure?

    a) The proximal port
    b) The distal port
    c) The inflation port
    d) The medial port

99. You will be assisting the physician with a Swan-Ganz insertion. What position should you place the patient in for this procedure?

    a) Left lateral supine position
    b) Right lateral supine position
    c) Fowler's position
    d) Trendelenburg position

100. Which medication can be administered through a bronchoscope?

    a) Topical lidocaine
    b) N-acetyl cysteine
    c) Fentanyl
    d) Aerosolized lidocaine

101. The typical pediatric dosage of fentanyl is:

    a) 0.05 mg/kg to 0.3 mg/kg with a max dosage of 0.4 to 0.6 mg/kg.
    b) 1 ug/kg to 3 ug/kg with a max dosage of no more than 5-10 ug/kg.
    c) 0.05 mg to 0.3 mg with a max dosage of 0.4 to 0.6 mg.
    d) 1 ug to 3 ug with a max dosage of no more than 5 to 10 ug.

102. Hypotonic saline is:

    a) Less viscous than hypertonic saline.
    b) More viscous than hypertonic saline.
    c) An example of a mucolytic agent.
    d) Used during routine endotracheal suctioning.

103. You notice that your patient's doctor has ordered a leukotriene modifiers as you are reviewing new physician orders for your 3 year old asthma patient. What would you do?

    a) Question the doctor about this order.
    b) Administer the drug using a nebulizer.
    c) Administer the drug with a mask.
    d) Ask the nurse to administer it.

104. Select the type of broncho-dilating medication that is accurately paired with an example of it.

    a) Ultra short acting bronchodilator: Albuterol
    b) Intermediate acting bronchodilator: Racemic
    c) Long acting bronchodilator: Salmeterol
    d) Ultra short acting bronchodilator: Pirbutrol

105. Which of the following inhaled respiratory medications can be taken without a spacer?

    a) Beclomethasone
    b) Budesonide
    c) Fluticasone propionate
    d) Triamcinolone acetonide

106. Your infant patient will be given natural surfactant. What should you know about natural surfactant, as the respiratory therapist?

    a) Natural surfactant is derived from stem cells.
    b) Natural surfactant is not as effective as synthetic surfactant.
    c) Children with congenital heart disease do not get natural surfactant.
    d) Natural surfactant is derived from bovine lungs.

107. Which infant is most likely to be a non-responder to surfactant treatment?

    a) An infant with altered surfactant metabolism
    b) An infant with an altered surfactant quantity
    c) An infant with pulmonary hypoplasia
    d) An infant with a gestational age more than 25 weeks

108. Which pediatric medication should be included in the pediatric crash cart?

    a) Atropine 0.5 mg/ 5 ml syringe
    b) Sodium Bicarbonate 5 mEq/10 ml syringe
    c) Sodium Chloride 0.45% 10 ml flush syringe
    d) Sodium Bicarbonate 3 mEq/10 ml syringe

109. T piece resuscitation devices are:

    a) More effective than a self-inflating bag resuscitator.
    b) Less effective than a self-inflating bag resuscitator.
    c) As effective as a self-inflating bag resuscitator.
    d) No longer used.

110. You are caring for a toddler in the emergency department. The child swallowed a bottle of aspirin. Which complication of this poisoning may this toddler most likely to be affected with?

    a) Respiratory acidosis
    b) Respiratory alkalosis
    c) Metabolic acidosis
    d) Metabolic alkalosis

111. You are assessing a toddler who has a barking like cough. Which disorder would you expect this child to have?

    a) Laryngotracheobronchitis
    b) Paralysis of the vocal cord
    c) Tracheitis
    d) Epiglottitis

112. Which patient is most at risk for vocal cord paralysis?

    a) A male patient
    b) A female patient
    c) A singer
    d) A concrete worker

113. Paralysis of the vocal cords:

a) Most often affects the left vocal cords.
b) Most often affects the right vocal cords.
c) Is most often bilateral.
d) Can be life threatening when it is unilateral.

114. Which patient is at greatest risk for retropharyngeal abscesses?

a) A preterm infant
b) A neonate with a surfactant deficit
c) A 4 year old child with asthma
d) A 4 year old child with a sinus infection

115. Which congenital disorder is characterized by a small oropharynx and a small mandible?

a) Choanal atresia
b) Subglottic stenosis
c) Pierre Robin Syndrome
d) Laryngomalacia

116. Select the congenital anomaly that is accurately paired with its possible treatment.

a) Choanal Atresia: Oral airway
b) Pierre Robin Syndrome: Supine positioning
c) Subglottic Stenosis: None. It is self-limiting.
d) Laryngomalacia: Surgical repair

117. The defining criterion for apnea of prematurity are:

a) Respiratory pauses of more than 20 seconds or an airflow interruption and respiratory pauses more than 10 seconds with bradycardia of less than 80 BPM

b) Respiratory pauses of more than 20 seconds or an airflow interruption and respiratory pauses more than 20 seconds with bradycardia of less than 60 BPM

c) Respiratory pauses of more than 20 seconds or an airflow interruption and respiratory pauses more than 20 seconds with bradycardia of less than 80 BPM

d) Respiratory pauses of more than 10 seconds or an airflow interruption and respiratory pauses more than 20 seconds with bradycardia of less than 80 BPM

118. About what percentage of premature infants have apnea of prematurity?

a) 10%
b) 15%
c) 20%
d) 25%

119. Which fact about apnea of prematurity is accurate?

a) It does not occur until about 14 days after birth.
b) It occurs about two or three days after birth.
c) It typically occurs immediately after birth
d) The central type of apnea of prematurity is the most common.

120. Which part of a pulmonary artery catheter hemodynamically determines cardiac output by comparing the difference between the pulmonary artery and the right atrium of the heart?

a) The distal lumen
b) The proximal lumen
c) The balloon inflation port
d) The thermistor

121. **Select the hemodynamic measurement that is accurately paired with its normal value.**

    a) Central Venous Pressure: 1 to 8 mm Hg
    b) Cardiac Output: 2 to 7 L/min
    c) Mixed Venous Oxygen Saturation: 40% to 80%
    d) Right Atrium Pressure: 2 to 15 mm Hg

122. **Your neonatal patient will be assigned what score, according to the Children's Coma Scale, when the infant has fixed pupils, paralyzed extra-ocular movement, spontaneous respirations and flaccid muscles?**

    a) 2
    b) 3
    c) 4
    d) 5

123. **Which law of physics states that the greater the cardiac preload that is in the heart's ventricle during the relaxed phase, or diastole, the greater the amount of blood of blood that will be moved from the heart during systole, or the contraction phase of the cardiac cycle, with other factors remaining constant?**

    a) Boyle's law
    b) Dalton's law
    c) Frank-Starling law
    d) Poiseuille's law

124. **Which form of pneumonia tends to be the most severe?**

    a) Viral pneumonia
    b) Bacterial pneumonia
    c) Fungal pneumonia
    d) Protozoan pneumonia

125. **Which is a risk factor associated with asthma?**

    a) Prepubescent female gender
    b) Post-pubescent male gender
    c) Asian ethnicity
    d) Second hand smoke

126. **Which pulmonary disorder is associated with paradoxical chest movement?**

    a) Pulmonary hypertension
    b) Flail chest
    c) Atelectasis
    d) Cardiac tamponade

127. **The normal urinary output for an infant is:**

    a) 5 to 10 mL/hr
    b) 10 to 20 mL/hr
    c) 0.5 to 5 mL/kg/hr
    d) 5 to 10 mL/kg/hr

128. **You are teaching a young mother about her neonate's nutritional needs. Which should be included in the teaching plan?**

    a) The neonate needs 2.25 to 4 g/kg per day of protein
    b) The neonate needs 60 kcal/kg/day for the first 3 months
    c) The neonate needs 100 to 120 mL/kg per day of fluids
    d) The neonate's diet should contain 70% of the diet from carbohydrates

129. **You are caring for an infant who is receiving hyper-alimentation to meet their nutritional needs. Which complication may this infant most likely to be affected with?**

    a) Respiratory acidosis
    b) Respiratory alkalosis
    c) Metabolic acidosis
    d) Metabolic alkalosis

130. **Which respiratory disorder has a characteristic "thumb sign" that can be seen with a lateral x-ray?**

    a) Foreign body aspiration
    b) Peritonsillar abscess
    c) Tracheitis
    d) Epiglottitis

131. Which of the following disorders is the most serious?

    a) Tracheitis
    b) Pertussis
    c) Retropharyngeal abscess
    d) Paralysis of the vocal cord

132. Which patient is least likely to be diagnosed with an MRI?

    a) An emaciated patient with possible pulmonary hypertension
    b) A morbidly obese patient with possible pulmonary hypertension
    c) An emaciated patient with a possible disorder of the major vessels of the heart
    d) A patient with a possible disorder affecting mediastinum

133. Pediatric apnea monitor alarms are typically set at:

    a) A cardiac rate of less than 80 per minute and more than 210 per minute as well as 15 seconds of apnea.
    b) A cardiac rate of less than 80 per minute and more than 150per minute as well as 15 seconds of apnea.
    c) A cardiac rate of less than 60 per minute and more than 150per minute as well as 20 seconds of apnea.
    d) A cardiac rate of less than 80 per minute and more than 150per minute as well as 20 seconds of apnea.

134. Polysomnography monitors and measures:

    a) Cardiac rate, O2 saturation, brain activity, eye movements, respirations, muscle tone and activity while the patient is experiencing narcolepsy.
    b) Cardiac rate, O2 saturation, brain activity, nasal flaring, respirations, muscle tone and activity while the patient is experiencing narcolepsy.
    c) Cardiac rate, O2 saturation, brain activity, hyper-resonance, eye movements, respirations, muscle tone and activity while the patient is asleep.
    d) Cardiac rate, O2 saturation, brain activity, eye movements, respirations, muscle tone and activity while the patient is asleep.

135. How much dextrose 5% is typically administered intravenously to neonates weighing less than 1500 gm?

a) 60 to 80 mL/day
b) 60 to 60 mL/kg/day
c) 60 to 80 mL/kg/day
d) 60 to 60 mL/day

136. Branched-chain ketoaciduria can be corrected with:

a) Kidney transplantation
b) Liver transplantation
c) A diet high in branched-chain amino acids
d) Low doses of glucose

137. Which fact about necrotizing enterocolitis should be discussed with the parents of the infant you are caring for?

a) Necrotizing enterocolitis primarily affects premature infants.
b) Necrotizing enterocolitis is rare among neonates.
c) Necrotizing enterocolitis occurs most often during the 6th to 8th month of life.
d) Necrotizing enterocolitis occurs most often with premature rupture of the membrane

138. Select the type of SMA that is correctly paired with its description.

a) Type I SMA: This type has an adult onset.
b) Type II SMA: Some children can have spontaneous recovery.
c) Type III SMA Werdnig-Hoffmann disease
d) Type IV SMA: Wohlfart-Kugelberg-Welander disease

139. You are caring for a young child who as scoliosis. The degree of the curve is 15 degrees. What should you discuss with the parent of this child?

a) Only angles greater than 40 degrees are of concern.
b) Only angles greater than 30 degrees are of concern.
c) Only angles greater than 20 degrees are of concern.
d) This is of concern, because the angle is greater than 10 degrees.

140. You are caring for a 7 year old ventilator dependent child in the home. The child also has home tutors. His grades are not good and he is not fond of school. Recently, he has taken an interest in piano lessons and is doing quite well with piano. What psychological defense mechanism is this child most likely demonstrating?

   a) Avoidance
   b) Approach-avoidance
   c) Compensation
   d) Sublimation

141. The purpose of guilt is to help the person to:

   a) Change behavior.
   b) Make amends.
   c) Prepare for death.
   d) Seek forgiveness.

142. Two of Engel's phases of grieving are:

   a) Anger and denial.
   b) Denial and acceptance.
   c) Restitution and developing awareness.
   d) Developing awareness and bargaining.

143. You are part of the hospice team who is visiting a mother after the death of her child from muscular dystrophy. The mother has now begun to withdraw from others and begin to restore her emotional wellbeing. Which phase of bereavement, according to Sander, is this mother in?

   a) Awareness of the loss
   b) Conservation
   c) Renewal
   d) Shock

144. Despite your urgings, the mother of an adolescent female at the end of life is not telling the girl about the terminal nature of her illness. How would you define this withholding of this information?

    a) Mutual pretense
    b) Illegal
    c) Psychologically neglectful
    d) Closed awareness

145. As you are caring for a patient in their home, the smoke alarm starts sounding and you notice a fire in the kitchen from the electrical outlets as well as in a frying pan filled with grease. What type of fire extinguisher should you use?

    a) Type A
    b) Type B
    c) Type C
    d) Type ABC

146. Which mnemonic is used to remember the correct procedure for using a fire extinguisher?

    a) RACE
    b) PASS
    c) FAST
    d) SWEEP

147. The triage color that is used for patients with nonthreatening injuries during an external disaster is:

    a) Red
    b) Yellow
    c) Green
    d) Black

148. Which of the following is a well-phrased learning objective?

    a) The RT will teach the patient about tracheostomy self-care.
    b) The RT will demonstrate the proper use of an incentive spirometer.
    c) The patient will learn about tracheostomy self-care.
    d) The patient will demonstrate the proper use of an incentive spirometer.

149. **What position does an infant assume when they are experiencing a "tet" spell?**

    a) A spread eagle position with flaccidity
    b) Complete adduction
    c) A knee to chest position
    d) Complete abduction

150. **Your patient has tracheomalacia and a cystic hygroma. What type of tracheomalacia does the patient most likely have?**

    a) Type I
    b) Type II
    c) Type III
    d) Type IV

ANSWER KEY

1.	C
2.	B
3.	D
4.	D
5.	B
6.	D
7.	C
8.	C
9.	D
10.	A
11.	B
12.	A
13.	B
14.	C
15.	C
16.	B
17.	B
18.	C
19.	A
20.	B
21.	B
22.	A
23.	D
24.	C
25.	B
26.	A
27.	D
28.	A
29.	C
30.	D
31.	C
32.	B
33.	C
34.	B
35.	D
36.	D
37.	B
38.	C
39.	B
40.	D
41.	C
42.	B
43.	D
44.	C
45.	D
46.	A
47.	C
48.	B
49.	C
50.	A
51.	C
52.	A
53.	D
54.	A
55.	A
56.	C
57.	B
58.	C
59.	A
60.	D
61.	A
62.	A
63.	C
64.	D
65.	C
66.	A
67.	B
68.	C
69.	D
70.	A
71.	C
72.	D
73.	B
74.	D
75.	D
76.	A
77.	C
78.	B
79.	C
80.	A
81.	D
82.	B
83.	D
84.	B
85.	B
86.	A
87.	D
88.	A
89.	A
90.	D
91.	A
92.	A
93.	A
94.	C
95.	B
96.	B
97.	C
98.	B
99.	D
100.	B
101.	B
102.	C
103.	A
104.	C
105.	A
106.	D
107.	C
108.	A
109.	C
110.	B
111.	A
112.	B
113.	A
114.	D
115.	C
116.	A
117.	C
118.	D
119.	B
120.	D
121.	A
122.	C
123.	C
124.	B
125.	D
126.	B
127.	C
128.	A
129.	C
130.	D
131.	A
132.	B
133.	A
134.	D
135.	C
136.	B
137.	A
138.	B
139.	D
140.	C
141.	A
142.	C
143.	B
144.	D
145.	D
146.	B
147.	B
148.	D
149.	C
150.	B

Made in the USA
San Bernardino, CA
10 March 2020

65520230R00226